CO

DISCLAIMER

This work is intended to supplement, **not replace** the advice of a trained health professional. The author specifically disclaims any liability, loss, or risk, personal or otherwise, that is incurred as a consequence, directly or indirectly of the use and application of any of the contents of this book.

ISBN: 9798300322557

Book cover created by J.J., the author of *The Internal Dragon: The Art of Self -Mastery*

Preface by LIQUID METAL

This is Dr. Bernard's work based on a reprint version. The original version must have been written before the year [1965] of his passing. I have two versions reprinted from other sources, and that's what prompted me to put together a book that is printed in a better readable book format. The ones I have are spiral notebook/typewriter format versions. I am an avid reader and book collector, so I took it upon myself to put together a proper book format version.

All credit and honor for the content (25 chapters plus Foreword page) **of "The Creation of the Superman" is Dr. Raymond W. Bernard's, the original creator of "The Creation of the Superman" knowledge/insight.**

Only the preface, end notes, images are created with an app (used for visual effect), a few interjections throughout the chapters and the commentary at the end of each chapter texts are my own words. The bio section texts, are research from various online sources. Whether the texts are unchanged from Bernard's original (6 decades ago) work or not, I do not know. We are in 2024 (at the time of this writing) and Dr. Bernard passed away 60 years ago. I'm just a person trying to bring awareness to Bernard's work. I could easily create a version based off his work, but I wanted to leave his words intact. Not many people know about Dr. Bernard's work, and that's what enticed me to dedicate some time in creating a book version so that more people are exposed to this common sense and yet esoteric important knowledge.

Knowledge is free, including everything written in this or any other book. You can find all knowledge for free, online or within yourself. But not everyone has the time to research all day for any given topic. And that's where authors come in. When you purchase books, you pay for the authors' time they have spent putting the book together. Knowledge is free, it was always and it will always be free. I put a good amount of personal time to put together this book in an easy and readable format.

I am not an author myself, but I write a lot on social media. This book is just a side project that I wanted to accomplish for the purpose of spreading truth about the importance of sexual continence i.e. conserving our sexual energy, raw food diet and honoring Dr.

Bernard. Whether something is true or not, it depends on the level of each individual's wisdom (experiences and knowledge). My intention is for Dr. Raymond W. Bernard's knowledge based on his research and life experience to reach a wider audience. In this world of chaos, suffering and terror, knowledge and insight is needed if we want our society to live in peace/harmony and prosperity. This was a huge task for me and I might not attempt to put together another book (personal creation) as I am very busy with other things in life. Hopefully this book helps you research and read more books by Dr. Bernard.

Note to men: In this book, among other subjects, there is something very important that Dr. Bernard wrote which may trigger you, and that is the "Parthenogenesis" subject. If it triggers you, it means that you are still in that extreme patriarchal mindset. The sooner you realize the importance of divine feminine, the sooner your divine masculine will emerge.

Note to women: Speaking of the same subject that may trigger men, if you are not in your divine feminine mindset yet, you may feel good about that subject and perhaps you may develop dislikement or hate toward men. I have personally met women that began hating men as soon as they read that they could have children without any men's spermatozoa. But they ran with their thoughts without realizing that women could bare children through parthenogenesis, will bear male children also, not just females. Both children must bond with both parents. In the case of male children, they need to bond with their father also. How would they become men without a masculine presence? Just read, without believing anything. Arouse your mind with curiosity.

Initially I wasn't even going to add anything at the end of each chapter and then I decided to add one or two paragraphs but eventually I added much more. Anything I write at the end of each chapter, you can use as you wish, you can copy and do with it as you please. We don't even know if our thoughts are really ours. Plus, nobody owns knowledge. Knowledge belongs to everyone. Don't let legality taint your moral compass. Say what you have to say, do what you have to do with a genuine intention to bring health, prosperity and happiness to the world.

I found it necessary to add some of my own thoughts at the end of each chapter. The chapters contain subjects that may trigger some readers. The commentary by me may also trigger people. Triggering is good, it helps us reflect on our beliefs.

In our modern world, with so much inverted and false information that we have, we are conditioned to believe something without taking in consideration that information that is different from what we believe may hold some truth to it. Not that what I write is the truth. It is up to each individual's consciousness at the current moment of their life to decide whether what they read resonates from their innermost being or whether it is their mind that tells them what to think.

Sometimes, very rarely, I may interject at the end of a paragraph or anywhere in the chapter and put some more context about what Dr. Raymond is saying so that some readers can have a better idea. One example is when Dr. Raymond says that fasting is not needed, unless what you need to live in complete health, is to receive all nourishment from the atmosphere/ether. Without context, some readers may be confused, since fasting has gained so much momentum in the recent times, but Dr. Raymond was speaking about bretharianism without mentioning the word "bretharianism". Any interjection by me, will be in parenthesis and accompanied by "L.M" or "Liquid Metal", as I don't want to put my words in Dr. Raymonds mouth. I am only responsible for what I think, say and do.

- Liquid Metal

CREATION OF THE

SUPERMAN

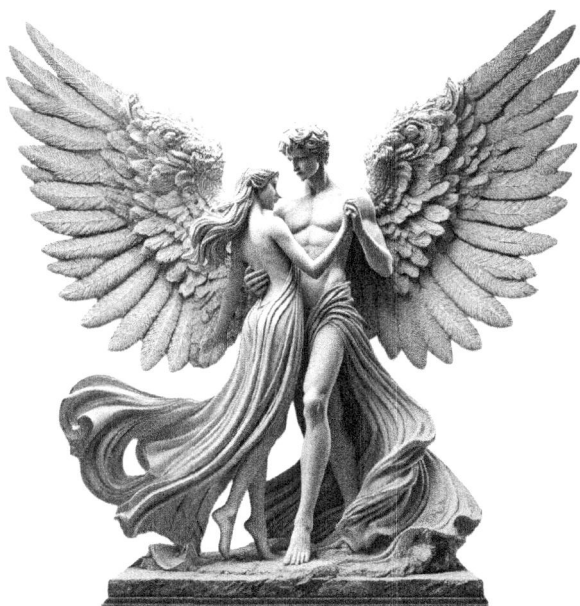

Dr. RAYMOND W. BERNARD

FOREWORD

The creation of the "Superman" was the original ideal behind all the great religions of the world in their original purity, before they were perverted and degenerated into ecclesiasticism. Examining the original doctrines of Brahmanism, Buddhism, Zoroastrianism, Orphism, Jainism, Taoism etc., we find running through them the golden thread of a Universal Religion, which we call Biosophy, the Science of Living.

Among these universal doctrines are Ahimsa (Non-Violence), Vegetarianism, Pacifism, Continence, Parthenogenesis (Virgin Birth) etc. It is the purpose of the following pages to elucidate these basic doctrines of human regeneration.

The founders of the great religions of Brahmanism (Chrishna), Buddhism (Gautama Buddha), Zoroastrianism (Zoroaster), Mayan Religion (Quetzalcoatl), Essenian Chrishnaism or Original Christianity (Apollonius of Tyana) were all eugenically created supermen, produced by parthenogenesis (without any male parent) and who enjoyed chaste gestations and lactations and painless childbirths.

The aim of these supermen was to teach humanity the laws of natural living and higher reproduction, whereby many more supermen like themselves may come into being. They all taught an identical teaching: practical methods for the attainment of individual and racial perfection. They all had the same objective: the conscious creation of a race of supermen. They were scientists, hygienists and eugenists of their day. But this scientific teaching was invariably perverted by the clerical founders of ecclesiasticism and the religious institutions founded on the basis of their teachings, which they degenerated and from a living organism became a dead and decaying carcass.

That is why many successive prophets and new religions were necessary, to restate, in their original purity the identical Biosophical Doctrines of Human Regeneration which were taught by their predecessors but which had since degenerated into a supernaturalistic ecclesiastical system both incomprehensible and impractical because not founded on natural law. What was once Biosophy and Science became Theology and Superstition, and light was replaced by darkness. As a result the race degenerated, and instead of evolving into supermen, degraded into submen. Meanwhile self-seeking priests concealed the truth, lest their own erroneous teachings may become too apparent through contrast.

Though suppressed and hidden for centuries, the Original Teachings that the churchmen opposed and did their utmost to destroy, the scientific and physiological doctrines of vegetarianism and continence are being rediscovered by scientific research which has brought to suffering, ignorant humanity, what degenerated false religions failed to bring. Such Biosophical research therefore stands on a higher level than existing religions and constitutes the nucleus of a New Scientific Religion of Hygienic and Eugenic Living, known as Biosophy. This new religion is not concerned with the worship of supermen of the past but in the creation of still greater ones to come.

Biosophy is a religion without imaginary man-gods, without messiahs and saviors, and without after-death heavens and hells. In place of multitudinous gods, products of the ecclesiastical imagination, who only tended to divide humanity into warring religious-racial factions and to promote planetary warfare, persecution and chaos.

Biosophy offers humanity a realistic, naturalistic and visible Creator in the form of the Sun, who is the God of science and the most ancient religions of Atlantis , Egypt etc. Who can deny that the Sun is the Universal Benefactor of the entire human race and the Giver of Life, not only to the plant, but to the human world as well? And in place of an imaginary heaven after death for departed souls, Biosophy offers a real Earthly Paradise to be enjoyed during this life. In fact, Biosophy is the first religion of the world to offer such an Earthly Paradise and to make its chief concern to make this life happy, healthy and long-extended, rather than bother about the after-death fate of the souls of its followers, while resigning them to a miserable existence during their lives.

Biosophy is a religion without bibles, without superstitions, without theologies, without dogmas, without churches, without priests, without foolish ceremonials, without supernaturalism, and without gods created from the imagination of priests for their own self-aggrandizement. Biosophy, on the other hand, is a religion founded on scientific research, on natural laws, on biological living, and on reason in place of blind belief or faith. It is a religion of Humanism, which is concerned with the betterment of humanity, and not with service to an imaginary and unreal god. Biosophy replaces gods by humanity as the objects of its service and replaces prayers by humanitarian and biological living.

Biosophy is a synthesis of seven Biosophical Sciences of Human Regeneration. These sciences are the following, The Biosophical Sciences of:

Agriculture
Nutrition
Bio-Therapeutics
Endocrinology
Eugenics
Anthropology
Cosmo biology

Through the application of these sciences, the Superman and the Super Race, which is the goal of Biosophy to create, will come into being. Since woman is the creator of the future race, the regeneration of the chalice for receiving the incarnation of higher beings, who require a superior method of conception (parthenogenesis), then alone can the CREATION OF THE SUPERMAN become a reality. How this may be achieved will be explained in the following pages.

> *"This work is dedicated to you, the living soul, the being who is created to live in eternal youth reality. You hold the key to beat aging and death. You are the elixir of life"* - Liquid Metal

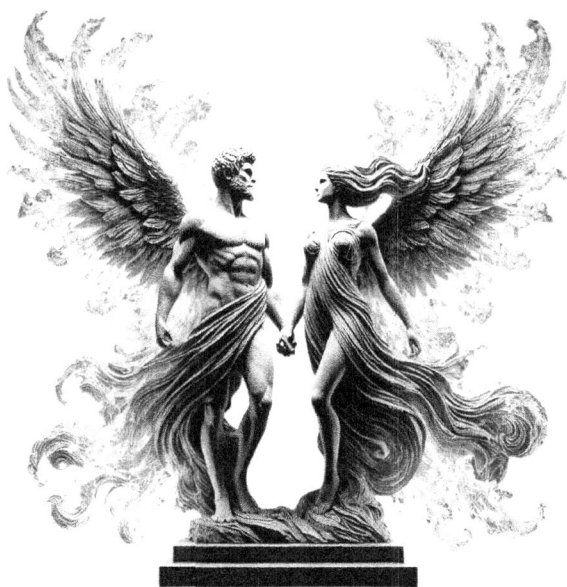

PART I

BIOSOPHICAL ENDOCRINOLOGY

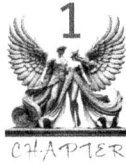

THE SEXUAL REGENERATION OF MAN: THE ELIXIR OF LIFE

MOST OF THE GREAT RELIGIONS OF THE WORLD were founded on one basic doctrine, the value of continence or chastity, usually exemplified in the immaculate sexual life, or rather non-sexual life of their founders, which was supposed to serve as a model for their followers. Coupled with this doctrine was that of Parthenogenesis of Virgin Birth, namely, that it is not necessary to commit the sexual act in order to render women fertile, so that continence may be practiced strictly and yet the race can continue.

While originally a Biosophical doctrine of human regeneration, the physiological value of continence later degenerated into a purely moral or ethical virtue, without hygienic significance; and finally became an exclusive attainment of a supernatural son of God, and hence impractical for most humans. As a result there developed a dualism of monastic orders claiming monopoly on this valuable physiological practice of sex hormone conservation, as part from the church goers, who were taught that they were natural sinners, and that the monks, by their austerity, vicariously atoned for their sins and so deserved their economic support. Through such false indoctrination, religion became a means of spreading vice and moral degeneration, rather than chastity.

With the decadence of the old religions, Biosophy is destined to rise as a New Religion based on a scientific conception of the physiological value of continence as a conservation of valuable sex hormones whose loss is depleting and harmful to body and brain and conservation beneficial. Dr. J.R. Brinkley., eminent endocrinologist, expresses the physiological reasons for sex hormones conservation as follows:

"I have not swerved from my original conception that the source of all human energy is sex energy, which is another way of saying that the glandular system of man is a chained system of series of connecting loops, mutually assisting or depressing each other by their secretions, of which series the genital glands seem to have the power of most directly stimulating and in a measure dominating the human body and mind by their particular kind of hormones, manufactured by the sex glands and distributed by the blood stream for the nourishment of all the tissues of the body".

An English physician, Dr. Knaggs, writes on this same subject:

"Strict continence enables the essence of these sexual secretions to be re-absorbed into the body. This not only makes for health but also build up those creative intellectual and intuitive faculties which show themselves in the work we do. Moreover, when we have learned to control this reproductive function, to turn inwards the mighty forces which it represents, we have solved one of the important problems of existence which brings us nearer to that superhuman stage to which we must ultimately attain".

The medieval alchemists were really endocrinologists and the Magnus Opus which they sought was not the artificial creation of gold out of lead but the sublimation and refinement of sexual energy, when denied a lower outlet into higher brain power through the ascent of the Kundalini Force from the pelvis to the brain. The conservation and transmutation of this vital force was their Elixir of Everlasting Youth and the secret of physical immortality for which they sought.

In our own day, modern physiologists have engaged in a similar quest. Several decade ago, Brown Sequards, the great French physiologist, put forward the assertion that the main cause of old age was a diminution in the quantity of absorbed seminal fluids (the internal sex secretion) present in the blood; and that its cure depended upon enriching the blood with this secretion. This he thought could be accomplished by a cutaneous injection of the spermatic fluid of an animal.

He failed to realize that a hygienic and continent life will cause the individual's own sex glands to be reawakened. The "Brown Sequard Elixir", however, proved ineffective, for it produced only a temporary invigoration. The next step in this direction was the direct implantation of animal sex glands into the human organism. But this "glandular grafting" of Dr. Voronoff, though it resulted in a longer stimulation, did not effect a permanent cure. If an old man may be temporarily rejuvenated by the implantation of the testicles of a goat or a monkey, surely he would have never grown old if he had retained his own in a normal condition by a continent life.

Senility, which is a product of sterility, or impotence, is an after effect of persistence sexual indulgence. The grafting of animal glands, like the Brown-Sequard spermatic injection, is a temporary, ineffective and fallacious method of rejuvenation, which does more harm than good. Weak genital glands, like any other weak part of the body, may be brought back to their normal state by the conservation of their secretions and by the purification of the blood through a natural diet.

The esoteric doctrine of the Eternal Life did not refer to the future existence of the soul in heaven, but to the present immortality of the physical body on Earth. Immortality is to be obtained right now, in the physical world, by hygienic and continent living. The doctrine of resurrection meant the transition from a mortal, decaying physiological state to an immortal, non-katabolic one. Most of us are walking around half dead. Four-fifths of our brain cells are inactive as a result of having been poisoned by injurious foods. By rejuvenating the body through obedience to the laws of nature, we may be raised from the dead, we may be resurrected.

The disease of senility may be permanently cured. Death is not a sudden occurrence, it is the termination of a slow process of dying. This dying, or cellular disintegration, may commence at birth; it is hastened by eating decaying dead food and by losing seminal fluid. This fluid, when retained within the body, becomes the elixir of eternal youth. When a man loses his seed in generation or sex indulgence, he throws away his creative substance, and in so doing, hastens death. He may not know the reason for the consciousness of the uncertainty of life, and the fear of death that is ever with him, but it is there with the average person, if he is honest and will admit it. This state of consciousness is caused by the loss of life, the life which should be retained within the body for its own health and increased vitality and the strengthening of the mind.

The sin of Onan, the waste of life-fluid was punished by death. This punishment was not an act of supernatural vengeance, but the physiological consequence of the loss of the power which animates the body. It does not occur suddenly but gradually. This gradual dying, which we call old age, is the natural result of sex indulgence. Gray hair is not to be venerated; it is a symbol of a wild and dissipated youth. One who lives as nature intended to live, in absolute chastity, will never grow old. Lifelong continence and a fruit diet will insure perpetual youth.

The old age is simply the product of weakened sex glands as a result of previous abuse, which is proved by the following statements by Dr. Voronoff;

"Decrepit old men are, in reality, "eunuchs". They have been emasculated. I have never known an eunuch to exceed the age of sixty. Well before death they have the appearance of old men, and from this, one might be tempted to attribute a very advanced age to them, but this would be a pure illusion. They have every appearance of being effectively aged; dry skin, bloated body and dull eyes. They have a stooping gait which gives one the impression that they are centenarians. Their death seem to be the normal end of old age, but verification of the facts usually indicates that they died between fifty and sixty years of age.

     Their aspect is the outcome of the fact that, deprived of the essential factor of youth and vigor, they have prematurely aged and have died well before the term ordinarily attained by normal men. Thus, then, the lack of the internal secretions from the sexual glands shortens life. It could not be otherwise; it is unthinkable that a body deprived of the organs, the suppression of which renders the blood poor, the bones frail, the muscles feebler, fat more abundant, nutrition imperfect, should not suffer a general enfeeblement, become more vulnerable and less able to struggle against the causes which always bring about death well before the normal physiological time".

"It may be affirmed then, that deprivation of the interstitial glands' internal secretion accelerates the advent of old age and shortens life. On the other hand, the maintenance of this source of vital energy is the best guarantee of longevity. Men who are endowed with active interstitial glands and in whom the functioning of these glands is not extinguished, lived to be very old"

In relation to the individuals of ancient biblical times, whose periods of life was supposed to have existed for more than a thousands years, the man of today is an eunuch who dies prematurely. The longevity of these prehistoric people was due to their fruit diet and to their lifelong chastity. Increasing incontinence, however, led to a gradual decrease in the length of life, until it extended for only a hundred and twenty-five years, and finally for only seventy years. Yet the human body was never supposed to decline or die, but to live forever, always increasing in youthfulness, strength and beauty. Old age and death, like disease, are the consequences of continued disobedience to nature's laws.

Metchnikoff considered the problem of old age from another point of view. He attributed senility to the fermentation and bacterial decomposition of waste matter in the intestines. He though that he found the elixir of youth in a fermented milk called "yogurt" which was supposed to contain bacteria that would counteract the toxic ones. However, he failed to realize that pathogenic bacteria may not thrive unless they have decaying matter on which to feed, which is provided for them when animal foods are eaten; and that a raw vegetable and fruit diet will keep the intestinal tract in a state of perfect purity.

Certain foods cause organic decay, while others prevent it. By eating only the latter (raw fresh vegetables and fruit), our flesh may be chemically preserved, and we may become living mummies. Aging results from a counterbalancing of anabolic (constructive) processes by katabolic (destructive) ones; and a raw fruit diet causes the former always to predominate, so that the tissues remain indefinitely as fresh and pure as those of an infant. Dr. Tilney, the neurologist says:

"There is strong argument in favor of the theory which holds old age in the brain, as in other organs, to be result of life's successive and cumulative intoxications. Old age in the brain is much more often the result of disease than of some inherent aging process".

Thomas Parr, who led a simple and unstimulating life in the country, subsisting on a natural diet, lived to be 152 years of age. His death was caused by the rich foods given to him when the King of England invited him to his palace. A post-mortem examination of his body made by Harvey, revealed the fact that his organs were in perfect condition, his sex glands being "large and voluminous". If he had continued his former way of living, there is no reason why he could not have reached his two hundredth year. On the island of San Salvador, a case was reported of a farmer who lived to be 180 years old. He also lived simply and chastely, eating only one meal a day, using meat very seldom, and fasting at regular intervals.

🔖 *Commentary by* LIQUID METAL

It is important to understand the difference between real religion and organized religion. The true religion cared about humanity, while organized religion suppressed humanity's potential and freedom. Religion in Latin is *'relegare'*, meaning to tie, to bind together. This has both a positive and a negative meaning. To tie together means to unite, but to tie or bind together means also to enslave, like tying someone's hand or their mind with invisible chains as in the case of the organized religion and the state.

Feel free to replace the term 'New Religion' that Dr. Bernard used, with 'Real Spirituality', where you are truly free of organized religion dogmas, free or government's tyranny and free of self-destructive beliefs.

When doctor Brinkley talks about the source of all human energy being "sex energy" to give you a hint as what that energy is, so that modern audience have a better understanding is that he is talking about the Kundalini energy. Also, when you read about continence, that means semen and ovum retention. The name of the book is the Creation of the Superman, but it means for both genders. Throughout this books you will read about avoiding certain foods completely and be chaste all life. Some information here may cause you to violently deny it, but check the title of this book, the word "Superman" (applies the same for women, "Superwoman) is in the title. There is a big difference between a strong man/woman and a superman/superwoman.

You may eat healthy (according to what you think healthy means) and exercise, and you may indeed be a strong man or a woman, but you will just add a few more years to your life compared to others. But becoming a superman or a superwoman, will add hundreds of years to your lifespan. If you don't believe this to be possible, it's because you either don't have the knowledge, or you know what needs to be done but you are still attached to man-made poisons (foods and drinks), attached to sex/lust and any other thing/habit that hold back your potential into becoming a superman or a superwoman.

Conserve your divine essence, it's how you become a superman or a superwoman, and not wasting it through procreation, conventional/ meaningless sex and pixels on the screen.

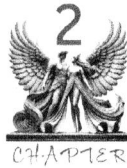

THE PHYSIOLOGICAL SUBLIMATION OF SEX ENERGY

UNDERDEVELOPED MEN AND WOMEN believe that sex is a plaything, something which no other purpose than to afford them amusement. But developed men and women know that this creative power has far more important uses than merely to be wasted in thoughtless indulgence. The sex glands are the engines of the human body, the generators of organic energy. This energy, if conserved, may become the motive power behind all accomplishments in life. The popular idea that most geniuses led immoral lives is false, as a study of their biographies proves. The reverse is rather the case, for creative ability, whether along artistic or intellectual lines, is a sublimated expression of the same vital energy which the average individual usually dissipates through sexual channels. Therefore, the supermen and the great geniuses of the past invariably led strictly continent lives.

The few talented individuals who did not, may not be classed among the spiritually highest. Their work lacks a certain subtle quality, which is present in a Beethoven symphony or in a painting by Leonardo da Vinci, that only results from a sublimation of sex energy.

The following celebrated individuals led strictly chaste lives:

Apollonius of Tyana (who, at the age of 20 said: "I am resolved never to marry, and to abstain from the company of all women whatsoever), John the Baptist and Jesus, greatest of prophets; Hypatia, Thomas Kempis, St. catherine of Siena, St. Theresa, Joan of Arc and Savonarola, greatest of mystics and martyrs; Pythagoras,

Plato, Aristotle, Thomas Aquinus, Francis Bacon, Spinoza, Leibnitz, Locke, Pascal and Kant, greatest of philosophers; Newton, greatest of scientists; Handel and Beethoven, greatest of composers; and Leonardo da Vinci, Michelangelo and Raphael, greatest of painters. The following great men lived continently during the creative period of their lives; Zoroaster, Moses, Buddha, St. Paul, Plutarch, St. Augustine, Dante, St. Francis, Erasmus, Descartes, Voltaire, Diderot, Milton, Schopenhauer, Nietzsche and Tolstoi.

The chastity of the supermen is due to physiological, not religious or theological reasons. These reasons, which constitute a body of new physiological facts of far greater importance than Harvey's discovery of the circulation of the deal with the origin and transformations of vital energy, and with the intimate relationships existing between the genital glands and the lymphatic , vascular and nervous systems. The human body is like a dynamo which draws its electric power directly from the ether.

> **“**
> Through lung and skin respiration, etheric power is absorbed into the body, collecting at the Solar Plexus, the battery of the sympathetic nervous system. From here, this electric energy (the Life Force) passes to the sex glands, where in combination with elements derived from the blood, it condenses into seminal fluid. **”**

(*Believe it or not, when you are not lustful anymore and when you have been conserving and transmuting your sexual energy through creativity, you stop producing seminal fluid. What I mean is that all the vital lifeforce circles back into the system unrestrained, it nourishes your body, mind and spirit; and anytime you want to have children, simply have sex and you'll be back to degenerating self-made reality, creating average offsprings. - L.M*)

It is through this secretion that vital energy is conveyed to the various ductless glands, nerve centers and organs of the body. From the ovaries (in males, the *testicle*), the sex secretion is carried by the Oviducts (in males, by the *vas deferens*) to the Uterus (in the male, the seminal vesicles). The latter organ, which acts as a seminal receptacle, is surrounded and permeated by a network of lymphatic vessels which absorb and draw up sexual fluid as quickly as it is being formed (in both sexes). This lymphatically absorbed seminal fluid is then collected at the Receptaculum Chyli, from where it is sent up through the Thoracic duct, into the left Subclavian Vein as it enters the heart. Thus it vitalizes the blood, giving it the capacity to transform inert food material into living tissue, and being carried by it to all parts of the body.

Through the Carotid Artery, the transmuted sex secretion is carried up by the blood to the brain, to nourish and energize its cells. In the Choroid Plexus of the Third Cerebral Ventricle, and in the Pituitary Body, it is transformed into cerebro spinal fluid and pituitrin, which flow through the cavity of the brain and spine, generating nerve electricity. It is for this reason that a persistent loss of seminal fluid, by causing a reduction in the quantity and concentration of cerebro spinal fluid, produces a devitalized condition of the nervous system, which we call "neurasthenia". Such consequences follow birth control practices.

Each night, during sleep, a new daily supply of cerebro spinal fluid is manufactured. Energy absorbed from the ether by the sympathetic nervous system (whose nerve-endings in the skin consist of minute mouths, which rhythmically open and close) is conveyed through the medium of the sex secretion to the central nervous system, which is then electrically recharged.

When this stored energy in the cerebro spinal fluid, after the day's activities is again expanded, a condition of drowsiness, or a desire for sleep ensues. It normally requires from three to five hours for this recharging of the central nervous system to take place; one should then immediately arise, for excessive sleep might cause the newly generated energy to be dissipated (through the uncontrolled cerebral activity of dreams).

It is through the medium of the sex secretion that the elements required for the nourishment of the cells of the brain and the nerves are transformed from their raw state, as obtained from food, to the vitalized condition in which they may be incorporated into nerve tissue. The sex glands are centers of phosphorus metabolism; they extract raw phosphorus from assimilated food, chemically transforming it (as their secretion), so that it may be absorbed and utilized by brain cells. If any of this vital fluid escapes (voluntarily or involuntarily), the blood is drained of phosphorus, and the brain is deprived of its nourishment.

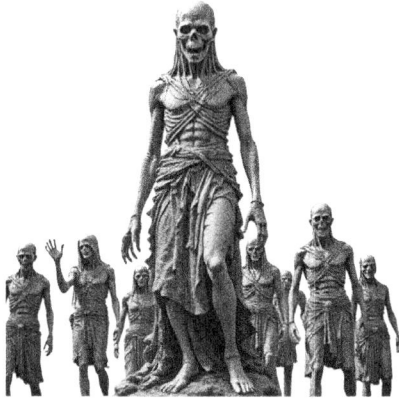

(*Most men and many women are "walking zombies" from too much seminal fluid wastage/expulsion through sexual intercourse, masturbations and orgasms.* - Ex-zombie, **Liquid Metal**)

Every drop of seminal fluid that is lost from the body brings disease, nervous derangement, mental decline, old age and death so much nearer to us. Until this loss of vital energy (in the females, the discharge of vaginal and uterine secretions, which is especially pronounced at the beginning and at the end of menstruation) is inhibited, one is like a leaking vessel, continually losing the Water of Life, and therefore, slowly dying. A seminal emission is the escape of incipient brain tissue.

Physiologists formerly thought that there were two separate sex secretions, an internal one produced by the interstitial cells and an external one, produced by the reproductive glands. This, however, was a false assumption – for the secretions of the genital glands (including the glands of the uterus and the seminal vesicles in addition to the ovaries and the testicles) constitute an indissoluble unit, all elements of which are continually being generated and lymphatically absorbed.

Spermatozoa and ova are not produced at rare intervals when required for reproductive purpose, but continually; they are absorbed by lymphatics into the blood stream, having an internal function to perform. Any escape of the seminal fluid involves a loss of the "internal secretion", which is nothing else than what has been called the "external secretion" when it is conserved, absorbed and physiologically utilized. There is really only one sex secretion, which is an internal secretion, the so-called external one being nothing else than a pathological escape of this.

Dr. Brinkley, the endocrinologist says:
"It is briefly my view that both the internal and external secretions of the gonads (sex glands collectively) are equally valuable to the upbuilding of body tissues, and that the gonads themselves are not merely a link in the chain of the endocrines. The gonads in the chain of the endocrines is the master position, and the well-being of all the endocrines is exactly dependent upon the well-being of the gonads. Defective thyroid glands can be most easily repaired by repair of the gonads, and so will all the glands of the chain".

The thyroid, pituitary and pineal gland, which are intimately related to the mental and spiritual life of the individual, are directly activated by the absorbed sex fluid carried to them by the blood. There is an intimate interdependence between the genital and the thyroid glands, as there is between the latter and the brain. A small thyroid secretion results in the development of a cretin, an idiotic dwarf, even as a diminished sex secretion produces an eunuch, an individual who is physically and mentally underdeveloped. At puberty, when a greater amount of sex secretion is sent into the blood, there is an increases thyroid secretion, accompanied by a rapid physical and mental development. On the other hand, when the sex secretion is lessened, as during senility, the thyroids shrivel, and a degeneration of body and mind results.

Dr. Voronoff writes: *"No organ can preserve its vital energy and function to full capacity if its cells are not stimulated and vivified by the genital glands' internal secretions. Eunuchs furnish a very clear demonstration of this. All their organs are like those of the rest of humanity, with one exception. Deprivation of this one organ depresses, weakens the functioning of all the others and brings premature old age. The removal of these organs reacts as much on the brain as on the heart, the muscles, the bones and all the other organs. The moral and physical energies both diminish. Abelard, the brilliant poet, never wrote a line after he was emasculated".*

Dr. Nicholas says: "It is a medical a physiological fact that the best blood of the body goes to form the elements of reproduction in both sexes. In a pure and orderly life this matter is reabsorbed. It goes back into the circulation ready to form the finest brain, nerve and muscle tissue. This life of man carried back and diffused through his system, makes him manly, strong, brave and heroic. The suspension of the use of the generative organs is attended with a notable increase of bodily and mental vigor and spiritual life. Nature finds another use for the unexpected sexual energy in employing it for the building up of a keener brain, and more vital and enduring nerves and muscles".

In the genital glands of animals and men there are secreted powerful and subtle chemical elements, which are absorbed into the blood and thence carried to all parts of the organism to energize, invigorate and strengthen the cells, organs and parts of the body, including the brain and nervous system. Some have gone so far as to hazard the opinion that old age is chiefly due to a lessening of the supply of these secretions.

Nature has ordained that all the secretions of the sex glands, in both male and female, be forever retained within the body, just as are the secretions of the other ductless glands. The sex glands are the only endocrine glands whose secretions may escape; and we must look here for the fundamental cause of glandular derangement with their accompanying pathological symptoms.

The normal development and well-being of body, mind and soul directly depends upon this absorbed sex fluid; and that is why an absolutely chaste life is the only healthy, natural and creative one. Moses said; *"If any man's seed of copulation go out from him, then he shall wash all his flesh in water, and be unclean until even"*, and Jesus taught: *"Whosoever is begotten of God doth not commit sin; for his seed remaineth in him"*.

Commentary by LIQUID METAL

At one point in this chapter, Dr. Bernard mentioned that excessive sleep might cause the energy stored to dissipate through the uncontrolled cerebral activity while you dream. Have you ever had a wet dream? Don't answers, I know you have. Everyone has. A wet dream is simply wasted stored energy. This energy (semen for men and vaginal/uterine discharges for women) contains phosphorus. "Phos" in Greek means   LIGHT. You are the LIGHT BRINGER, you produce your own Light or the elixir of immortality. Semen retention for men and ovum retention for women is a must for the rejuvenation of the body, mind and the nervous system. Anyone who ejaculates, voluntarily or involuntarily through dreams, or menstruates, is slowly dying. Keep reading this book until the end and you should have a broader understanding of what magnificent of created beings we are.

Whether you are a woman or a man, it doesn't matter, both sexes can have wet dreams, both men and women will ejaculate secretions. The less you are bombarded with sexual content or thoughts, the less chance for you to have wet dreams, especially in the last 2 hours before you go to sleep, your mind should not be distracted with anything sexual. It is important to go to sleep early and get up early. When the Sun is out, or when it is not anymore dark, the body must be awake. Or else the biological clock of the body begins to malfunction. Your body won't know when it is dark and when it is day. Just as when the fullness and hunger hormones are damaged where the body doesn't know when it is full and when it is hungry, you'll read a bit about this later on.

Speaking again of sleeping only 3-5 hours, when you wake up, plant positivity in you, write or say affirmations out loud or in your mind, go outside of the house and breathe in fresh air through your nose. Never breathe through your mouth. Only your nose's hair can clean up the air. But in the morning, the air is much cleaner. Don't rush to check your phone (social media). Begin the day with joy and happiness. Plant the seed of health and freedom. Your sexual energy must be saved at all cost.

> J.J., in his book, **The Internal Dragon: The Art of Self-Mastery** writes: "*Semen is considered the most refined energy within the body, a fluid that when conserved, has the power to nourish not only the physical body but also the spiritual body. Just as the Tree of Avalon draws its power from the earth and the heavens, so too does the practitioners draw on their life force to fuel their spiritual ascent. In Druidic alchemy, the preservation of semen is a process of concentration and sublimation – the process by which the base elements of the body are refined and transformed into higher spiritual energy. This transformation mirrors the alchemical process or turning lead into gold, or more accurately, base consciousness into divine enlightenment*".

Taurus rules the thyroid gland, regardless of which zodiacal sign you may be. If you have any problem with thyroid consume peppers, pumpkins, spring onions, lentils, leeks, celery.

Scorpio rules the genitals, anus, urethra and prostate. foods to consume more than other foods for genital health: Lentils, turnips, cucumbers, cauliflower, onions, Brussel sprouts.

Each zodiac constellation controls certain parts of the body. You are all zodiacal signs. You might have heard of the constellation Ophiuchus. It is recognized as the 13th constellation but not an actual main zodiacal sign.

"Health must be a combinations of foods, Sun, exercise, meditation, grounding [barefoot walk on grass/soil/sand], conscious breathing, gratitude/appreciation, sexual energy conservation and transmutation, love etc. Complete health means not just physical but also mental, emotional and spiritual. Many people spend a lot of money on organic food and they still have health problems. There's much more to health than just what we eat. But the foods under your Sun sign are very important to be consumed regularly. It is a MUST. Let's suppose that you are Sagittarius.

The Cell Salt mineral that you are deficient of is "Silica". But it doesn't mean that you cannot be deficient of any of the other 11 Cell Salts. It is less likely but it is possible. If you barely consume raw fruit and vegetables where most of your diet is pasta, pizzas, crackers, ice cream or many other man-made processed so-called foods-drinks, you could be deficient of other Cell Salts. The term "being healthy" means different things to different people. What is healthy and what tastes good are two different things. Processed foods/drinks, alcohol, ejaculating, porn, conventional sex without genuine intention are some of the things that people are attached to.

These things are seen as being healthy to many people. Health is when you feel optimal in physique, mind, emotions and spirit. How many people do you know that are fully healthy? I know nobody. Everyone is deficient of something, be it Cell Salts, love, care, thoughtfulness etc." – page70, **TO BE REBORN** by Tamo A. Replica

Information such as in this book helped me understand better myself. I have children, and definitely they are not supermen, but they and yours can become. Too much excessive seminal emissions throughout my life up until 10 years ago, drained me of my life force which in turn affected my children and myself. I have been working hard on gaining back my true self since then. You are still early on in this book, after you read the whole thing, then you should have a better perspective on everything you need to know about your life and reality in general. Understanding our own mistakes is the beginning of the great path. And to understand ourselves, the first step is to stop lying to ourselves. The more we lie, the further we push the inevitable.

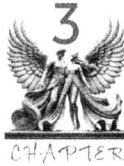

THE CAUSE AND CURE OF SEMINAL EMISSIONS

IN SPITE OF THE UNIVERSALITY OF THIS CONDITION and contrary to the orthodox medical teaching that it is normal, seminal emissions (in the female, leucorrhea, mucus discharges from the genital organ) are decidedly pathological. They have definite causes, and experience proves that once these are removed, they will disappear. They do not occur among animals and are unquestionably the results of unnatural living.

Nocturnal emissions are really a mild form of spermatorrhea, the male equivalent of leucorrhea. Leucorrhea is not the discharge of a lubricating fluid in the vagina, or of useless mucus, but of valuable seminal fluid, the raw material of brain-tissue (both of the maternal and the embryonic organism). This fluid is highly charged with electric energy, and its loss devitalizes the nervous system.

Involuntary seminal emissions occur in both sexes, the female being subject to much greater loss, in this respect than the male. That this condition is morbid is proven by the fact that its pathological after-effects are identical as those which follow its physiological analogues; masturbation and sexual intercourse. One subject to involuntary losses cannot claim to be leading a chaste life. Indeed, repeated seminal emissions involve a much greater loss of vital fluid than that caused by an occasional orgasm. The former condition is one of greater incontinence than the latter.

According to Mosaic Law, a male or a female subject to involuntary seminal emissions was considered as "Unclean (incontinent, or unhealthy), even as was one who indulges in sexual intercourse. To meat eaters this law may not seem rational, but to vegetarians, as were the followers of Moses, it is perfectly obvious. Seminal emissions are due to two fundamental causes:

1- **Wrong diet** (the eating of animal foods, eggs, dairy products and grains)

2- **Incontinence**

It is physiological fact that seminal emissions, in both male and female, may be caused and aggravated by sexual indulgence, and that a strictly continent life is the most important factor in their cure. They are not the escape of excessively produced semen, or of sexual energy, which was denied gratification, as was formerly supposed.

Almost all women are continually losing sexual fluid; the Water of Life is slowly escaping from their bodies. It is for this reason that woman is the "weaker sex", though the female organism should be as strong as the male (as it is among primitive people). This persistent loss of seminal fluid (especially at the commencement and at the end of each menstrual flow) results in the premature atrophy of the ovaries (the menopause), which is the direct cause of senility.

By retaining all genital secretions within the body, the ovaries may continue to function throughout life, and instead of the menopause and old age (which are the unnatural results of previous incontinent and unhygienic living), there will be perpetual youth and the indefinite retention of the reproductive capacity.

Previous sexual indulgence (either masturbation or its equivalent, sexual intercourse) produces a weakened and prolapsed condition of the sex organs, which induces seminal emissions. When one is in perfect health, and is leading a continent (chaste) life, all generated sexual fluid is immediately absorbed into the circulation where none of it is wasted. An internal obstruction to this lymphatic absorption and the subsequent overaccumulation of seminal fluid within its containers, may lead to its discharge.

Sleeping with a full bladder and rectum causes a compression of the seminal vesicles (or the uterus) which lie sandwiched in between them. This may result in an emission. All foods that are constipating, or which irritate the sexual nerve-centers, may cause seminal emissions. These include: *meat, fowl, fish, shell-food, eggs, dairy products, bread, cereals, cake, pastry, salt, pepper, spices, sugar, mustard, alcohol, tea, coffee, chocolate, candy and ice cream.* Because of their irritating and stimulating effects upon the sex organ (causing masturbation in children), these foods should be eliminated from the diet. By subsisting exclusively on raw vegetables and fruit, and by leading a continent life, one may forever do away with involuntary seminal losses. This conserved energy will then be transformed into mental and spiritual power.

The experiment of the American nutrition authority, Dr. Francis G. Benedict, on a group of 24 normal young college men, have shown that nocturnal emissions are products of the protein content of the diet. Putting these subjects on a low protein diet for 4 months, nocturnal emissions disappeared in most cases, to return again when the previous high protein meat diet was resumed. Benedict showed that not only nocturnal emissions but sex desire and all sexual phenomena are subject to dietary control, particularly the protein content of the diet. On a low protein diet, they disappear. This proves that sexuality in man is an abnormal effect of a high protein diet, and that chastity will become the rule when the diet is carefully regulated to be low in protein.

To cure seminal emissions, a total avoidance of erotic thoughts, reading, feelings, associations and practices is necessary. One must not smoke, for nicotine has a poisonous effect upon the sex organ and their secretions. Lascivious dreams are cerebral reflexes of our thoughts during the day; they may be prevented by a constructive direction of mental energies during waking hours. Incipient emissions during sleep may be, and should be, immediately inhibited and indrawn by a conscious effort of the will.

One should arise on first wakening no matter the time or how long one has slept, for emissions are most liable to occur towards the end of sleep (after dawn), when dreams are most prolific and when the bladder and colon being most distended, induce the greatest pressure upon the seminal vesicles or the uterus. The sexual organs, as well as the whole body, should be daily washed with cold water, especially on arising and before retiring. Sun baths are very beneficial, and sufficient outdoor exercise is advisable. It is best to sleep nude or in a night gown. Woolen underwear should not be worn, neither should a belt, for anything tight around the waist interferes with the lymphatic absorption of seminal fluid. It is best to avoid indoor occupations which compel one to be seated all day, and to engage in those necessitating outdoor physical activity.

Nothing should be eaten or drunk for several hours before retiring (before going to sleep). The largest meal should be at noon, not eating anything, except possibly fruit, in the evening. It is best to retire shortly after sundown, and to arise as soon after midnight as one first awakens, for emissions and lascivious dreams are less liable to occur before midnight than after. One should not sleep in a hotel, or on a mattress which has been promiscuously used. Neither should one sleep on a spring, or on a soft yielding surface. This causes the pelvic region of the body to sink downwards, which results in a congestion of the circulation in the genital region, a condition conductive to emissions. One should sleep outdoors, winter as well as summer, on a smooth, hard surface (such as a thin mattress placed on boards), using a pillow. It is best to sleep on the right side.

Commentary by LIQUID METAL

A book must test your will, your beliefs and rationality. If a book tells you to do what you'd like to do and if a book tells you not to do what you don't like to do, you will not grow. You mind cannot open from a room without windows. It's not just about books but also about people you have to deal with in life. Naturally, we don't like to be told what to do. But there is a big difference between someone that tells you (on your face or deviously) to do something for personal gain and someone whose intention is genuine to help you find your way. Don't think that everyone tries to get something out of you. There are people whose mission is to help the world become free.

I was the one that I never thought that seminal fluid could be contained. And I was wrong, I was consuming wrong foods and drinks, I was driven by lust. My sexual glands were over stimulated. But eventually, through hard work, I managed to retain my life force for good. You too, can conserve your sexual fluid, but you must put in the effort. If everything could be easily achieved we wouldn't grow spiritually. We would have remained adults in body but children in the mind.

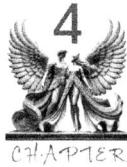

THE CURE OF MENSTRUATION AND THE PREVENTION OF THE MENOPAUSE

IT HAS BEEN SAID, *"Among all the inhabitants of the civilized world there is not one perfectly healthy woman"*. This is largely due to the fact that women have always been greatly miseducated and misled concerning matters of most vital importance to them. The traditional beliefs that a periodic flow of blood from the female genital organs, from puberty 'till the menopause, is a perfectly healthy, natural and necessary occurrence, that a sparse flow, or none at all, at the accustomed period, is a sign of bad health and that a woman who does not menstruate may not conceive, are utterly false and are contrary to physiological facts. Not very long ago, the medical profession thought that it was to a patient's advantage to draw off his "bad blood" by cutting a vessel, or by leeching. However, we now know that this is an injurious practice, for the blood is a homogeneous liquid.

What escapes is not "bad blood" but the fluid which vitalizes, nourishes and strengthens the body. In the same way, the old conception of menstruation as a purifying process has been discarded by the scientific world. Menstruation is a periodic hemorrhage of the female reproductive organs, resulting from certain definite causes whose removal will permanently do away with this abnormal loss of vitality.

Edward Carpenter, in his widely read book "Love's Coming of Age", says:

"There is little doubt that menstruation, as it occurs today in the vast

majority of cases, is somehow pathological and out of the order of nature. In animals, the periodic loss is so small as to be scarcely noticeable, and among primitive races of mankind it is as a rule markedly less than among the higher and later races. We may therefore suppose that its present excess is attributable to certain conditions of life which have prevailed for a number of centuries, and which have continually acted to bring about a feverish disposition of the sexual apparatus, and a hereditary tendency to recurrent manifestations of a diseased character. Among conditions of life which in all probability would act in this way may be counted:

1—The indoor life and occupations of women, leading to degeneration of the neuro-muscular system, weakness and inflammability.

2—The heightening of the sex passion in both men and women with the increase of luxury and artificialism in life.

3—The subjection of the woman to the unrestrained use and even abuse of the man, which inevitably took place as soon as she, with the changes in the old tribal life, became his chattel and slave, and which has continued ever since.

These three causes acting together over so long a period may well seem sufficient to have induced a morbid and excessive habit in the female organism; and if so, we may hope that with their removal, the excess itself and a vast amount of concomitant human misery and waste of life-power will disappear".

The universal shame and secrecy with which women regard menstruation, as they do any disease of the reproductive organs, indicates its pathological character. And we have only to observe the morbid symptoms which accompany menstruation to be convinced of the correctness of such a view, and that Moses was justified in classifying the menstruating woman together with the individual who lost seminal fluid, either involuntarily or through voluntary indulgence, as being "unclean". Most prominent of these symptoms relate to disorders of the heart and the vascular system. The loss of blood cause the heart to beat faster in order to pump the smaller quantity of blood through the body. This periodic overworking of the heart leads to subsequent cardiac trouble, for the heart was designed for a constant, not a variable quantity of blood in circulation. This results is a rapid and palpitating heartbeat, sudden flushings and pallors, strong pulsation in the carotid arteries (leading up to the brain) and a diminished hemoglobin-richness of the blood (anemia).

Menstruation is accompanied by a flow of blood to the genital organs, a pressure in the lower part of the belly, and a tenderness of the pelvic region. The mucous membranes of the labia and vagina become swollen, the clitoris becomes conspicuous, and a slight secretion appears in the genital passage. A condition of abnormal sensitiveness and irritability of the sex organs results.

As the menstrual flow is induced and augmented by sexual hyperemia, or vascular congestion in the uterus, so is this caused by wrong diet. As mentioned before, the mucous membranes of the vagina are similar to those of the nose, and as bad food (starches, sugars and animals food, which generate acid toxins in the blood) may lead to a catarrhal condition, a chronic mucous secretion, in the latter so may it cause emissions of vaginal and uterine mucous (seminal fluid). Leucorrhea is equivalent to a cold in the nose and is primarily due to wrong diet (as well as to sex indulgence).

In the male, a vicarious form of menstruation, through the nasal mucous membrane occurs. This is usually the after effect of seminal emissions, which in turn, are caused by bread and other mucus forming foods. We may express the relationship as follows:

(a)- **Wrong Food - Seminal emissions (leucorrhea or sexual orgasm)**

(b)- **Menstruation - The menopause - senility - death**

Menstruation may be reduced and finally done away with by the adoption of a hygienic diet. A certain girl, who possessed strength and vitality rarely seen among females, revealed the fact that since she began living on a fruitarian diet, her menstrual flow was reduced to barely a few drops, causing her not the slightest discomfort, nor preventing her from going bathing. Another girl, seventeen years of age, after adopting a vegetarian diet, did not menstruate for a year, during which time she was endowed with superior health, power and ability.

A friend of hers, who, in order to reduce, went on the same diet, did not menstruate for 6 months. However, since she was subject to the old medical superstition that the cessation of menstruation before the menopause is always pathological and dangerous, worry brought her to a nervous state. She went to a physician who attributed the cause of her trouble to menstrual suppression and forced menstruation through pills. (Thus are women misled and injured by false traditional conceptions).

When menstruation is cured, through the application of hygienic methods (which does not mean its suppression, but the removal of its cause), there will be no menopause, or atrophy of the ovaries, which results from the persistent loss of seminal anti menstrual fluids. The ovaries will then continue to function throughout life, and the reproductive capacity will be retained until a very advanced age, as is the case of Sarah, who gave birth to Isaac when she was ninety.

This is proven by recent experiments in the field of glandular radiation. We have been accustomed to believe that the menopause was an inevitable consequence of nature. "We now know that this is a false assumption. One New York doctor radiated a woman of 63 who had experienced her menopause at 46. At 64 the lady gave birth to a child" It is a known fact that excessive sexual intercourse, particularly when birth control measures are employed, may cause barrenness. The menopause, which is an unnatural condition of barrenness, may be cured by a natural diet and by the total conservation of seminal fluids. Senility and death may thereby be permanently prevented.

The uterus and vagina contain glands which produce a secretion in addition to that of the ovaries. The lymphatic vessel which surrounds these organs continually absorb this vital fluid for the enrichment of the blood and the invigoration of the nervous system. By living on a natural diet, and by keeping the body in a state of perfect health, no seminal fluid or blood will ever be discharged from the female sex organs.

"The uterus normally lies in a horizontal position, it's closed and tipping down, so that all of the glandular fluids within it may be retained. A distended bladder and rectum, however, will raise it to a vertical position, with the open end at the bottom, compressing it and squeezing out its contents. This uterine displacement (produced by constipation and by the wearing of a corset), in addition to the inflammation of the genital mucous membranes produced by toxins in the blood and by sexual intercourse, leads to leucorrhea, which in turn, causes menstruation"

It is very important that the digestive organs be kept scrupulously clean by living on a raw vegetable, fruit and nut diet. Other hygienic aids in overcoming menstruation are: sufficient outdoor exercise, deep breathing, the drinking of plenty of spring water, sun baths, cold sitz-baths and outdoor sleeping (on a smooth and hard surface). The secretions of the uterine, vaginal and Bartholin's glands, like those of the ovaries, have an important internal function; they should never be permitted to escape. This vital loss (either by orgasm, leucorrhea or mucous discharged at the menstrual period) devitalize the organism, leading to the premature atrophy of the ovaries (the menopause and senility).

The main cause of this mucous discharge from the vagina is wrong food. Its prevention depends upon the elimination of meat, chicken, fish, eggs, dairy products, white sugar, cooked foods, coffee, tea, salt, bread and cereals from the diet. By thus removing the dietetic cause of the discharge of uterine mucous, menstruation will automatically disappear.

Anything tight around the waist (a corset or belt) interferes with natural abdominal breathing (causing high chest breathing) congests the pelvic circulation and constricts the lymphatic ducts which carry up absorbed seminal fluid. Clothing, therefore, should be hung from the shoulders. The sex organs should not be overheated by being covered too much during the menstrual period. The full oxygenation of the blood, with pure air, reduces menstrual discharges.

Acids in the blood, resulting from the eating of meat, eggs, bread and sweets, makes it very thin and freely flowing, while an alkaline blood, rich in organic minerals obtained from raw vegetable and fruit, clots immediately on exposure to air. To cure menstruation, it is very important to adhere strictly to the raw vegetable, fruit and nut diet, eliminating all other foods. In addition to this, a strictly continent life in thought, feeling and action is necessary. In young girls, menstruation may be prematurely induced by erotic novels and motion pictures.

The following exercise, by strengthening the muscles of the uterus and the vagina, will aid in conserving seminal fluid, in curing menstruation and in insuring painless childbirth.

Exercise #1: Stand with your back to a vertical pole, or to the trunk of a tree. Then bend backwards, grasping the pole or tree with your hands, and descend as far down as you can go (going lower and lower each day, until your head finally touches the ground). By contraction of pelvic muscles, slowly rise to the original position. Follow this by deep abdominal breathing and repeat the exercise until the first signs of fatigue.

Hiram Butler, a pioneer in the field of teaching women how to overcome leucorrhea and menstruation, says:

"With many women the escape of the life fluid is almost imperceptible, so that only experience can teach her when she is fully conserving. There may be the frequent escape of, perhaps, only a drop at a time with no attending sensation. This is removed by the friction of the clothing; and so the escape of the life-forces goes on continually, and there is often a more thorough depletion than in the case of a person who loses by frequent orgasms. In many cases this gradual loss is the only way in which the life fluid escapes; in others, where the sex nature is active and life is generated rapidly, there may be at times, in addition to the gradual loss, an involuntary orgasm".

Women, therefore, have both these dangers to watch out for and overcome, the gradual loss of life fluid and a sudden loss through orgasm. The first step in this direction is, of course, to avoid sex stimulation by the opposite sex, whether in the form of kissing, embracing, petting, or more intimate sexual approaches. Strict continence should be the rule. Whenever a woman feels a slight tickling in her vagina, she should assume a horizontal position so as to prevent its gravitation pull downward, and practice contractions of the vaginal sphincter muscles. This will help her conserve the life fluid otherwise lost. To tone and strengthen these muscles, daily cold sitz baths plus exercises in muscular contractions are beneficial. Chastity in thought and act, adopting the horizontal (or better, the reversed position, with feet higher than the head) position, cold sitz baths and yoga exercises are the techniques for accomplishing this great work of female regeneration. Yoga postures in which the feet and pelvis are higher than the head are especially beneficial. And of course a low protein vegetarian diet is important, in fact all-important, in achieving the work of female regeneration.

Commentary by LIQUID METAL

Speaking of barrenness, to become fertile again, doesn't necessarily mean for the purpose of giving birth to more children. You may not want to give birth to children anymore, but the point of gaining back fertility is to gain back youthfulness and preventing aging. The same applies to men. Both men and women are designed to be fertile for hundreds of years if not forever. The elixir of immortality is within each one of us. In movies or in magazines etc. you may have seen the elixir of youth or the fountain of immortality they seek externally.

Those who don't know, seek it externally, those who don't want you to know, purposefully direct your attention to seek it externally without telling you that you are the fountain of youth. My friends, this is the ultimate secret, that you are immortal and that you can regain your immortality by being a serious practitioner of raw food consumption, fasting and anything else mentioned in this book. You may be a meat eater and may disagree, just as an alcoholic or a drug addict would disagree if you tell them that their choices are killing them from the inside. Just move on, when the time is right, everyone will come to the realization that to be alive, we must feed ourselves with life and not with death.

If you want change in your life, then change your habits. To become truly healthy we must give up everything this decaying system provides for us to be sick. Where it said that one of the aids is to drink spring water, it actually means water from an actual spring. Bottled water you purchase in stores that say "spring water" is not spring water. Nobody who cares about your health would package water in plastic bottles. If you have to buy the water, purchase water that is in glass bottles or jugs.

The next step to do, if bottled water in glass is not available or too expensive, then consume just homemade fruit juice. The cleaner your body becomes the faster you will rely on its own made water called "endogenous". When that time comes, you will not have to urinate anymore because the body is designed to function with the liquids and substances that it produces by default. There is a specific amount of blood and liquids that the body is designed to function in an optimal shape. But we have been consuming toxic foods and drink all life, therefore the body has been altered or broken, but it can be repaired when we do the great work through sheer will, determination and discipline.

When Dr. Raymond used the words "vegan and/or vegetarian" he means raw food. Any product labeled "vegan" bought in stores is poison. A lot of people don't see improvement from vegan products purchased in stores and they blame veganism. Raw fruit, vegetables, herbs, seeds and nuts equals "veganism", anything else is unhygienic.

PART II

REGENERATIVE
VS
DEGENERATIVE MARRIAGE PRACTICES

The truth about birth control

"To have intercourse for any other purpose than the procreation of children is to offer an insult to Nature. Marriage is the desire for the procreation of children, not the inordinate excretions of the seed, which is contrary to all law and reason" – Clement of Alexandria

"Among the higher classes, unrestrained sexual intercourse, for which the male and the marriage laws are responsible, leads to the practice of contraception and abortion. These practices, together with the sometimes-daily misuse of the female genitive organ by the male, lead to various diseases of that organ, common among which is cancer, and lead also to the ultimate perversion or destruction of the maternal instinct. If contraceptive methods, under the name of 'birth control' or any other name are taught to the majority of the woman of the masses, the race will become generally diseased, demoralized, depraved and will eventually perish". **– Thurston's Philosophy of Marriage**

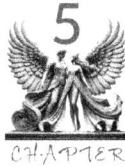

THE DANGERS OF CONTRACEPTION AND ABORTION

From a **Gynecological Point of View**.

THE BIRTH CONTROL MOVEMENT was initiated by Neo-Malthusian sociologists, by individuals who were not physicians, and who were ignorant of the physiological processes and the pathological consequences involved in what they were proposing. They thought in terms of the rise and fall of population in relation to the food supply, not in terms of vaginal and uterine pathology. To solve their sociological problems, they uncritically accepted a device whose physiological effects they had not investigated. In a matter of such importance, are we to be guided by sociologists, and by physicians who have been convinced by sociologists, or by specialists and experts on the subject, by gynecologists?

Gynecologists, above all others, have had an opportunity to study the effects of birth control measures upon the genital organs, especially those of women, and therefore, they have a right to pass judgment upon them. There is almost universal agreement among gynecologists that contraptions, as well as other methods of preventing conception, is decidedly injurious. We shall now review the opinions of twenty of the world's leading gynecologists on the subject of birth control. Their conclusions are based upon the observation of cases in which various methods have been used, principally coitus interruptus and contraception (both of which practices lead to similar pathological after-effects).

Dr. Giles, one of the foremost British gynecologists, says:

"When Birth Control is exercised from the outset of married life, and before any pregnancies have taken place, it seems certain that the practice favors the development of fibroid tumors of the womb".

"**Beard**, in his work on sexual neurasthenia, maintains that the sudden interruption of coitus (and also the use of condoms and similar practices) is not only far more deleterious than unduly frequent normal intercourse, but he point out that (in as much as, owing to the unnatural mode of sexual intercourse, the possibility of fertilization is almost completely prevented) sexual intercourse is apt, in such cases, to be indulged in far more frequently, and often to gross excess. More particularly in such circumstances are evil effects on the nervous system likely to ensue, since we have a combination of excessively prolonged and frequent sexual intercourse".

"**Dr. Kisch**, a German gynecologist, in his book, "*The Sexual Life of Woman*", says: "The most trustworthy method for the prevention of pregnancy is that of Malthus, permanent sexual continence. This recommendation, to which Tolstoi in the Kreutzer Sonata gives his adhesion, has recently found an advocate in a modified form in the distinguished gynecologist Hegar. The use of various measures for the prevention of conception is considered by Hegar to be harmful, at any rate in the case of young women. This practice gives rise to anemic conditions, and to nervous weakness and irritability".

Ribbing (another gynecologist) writes: "Although the sexual impulse is the product of a powerful developmental force, still the temporary and sometimes even the permanent control of this impulse is a moral civilizing force of enormous importance" The writer is opposed to the use of artificial preventive measures, he considers them untrustworthy and dangerous to health. Noteworthy, also, are the psychical considerations adduced by Ribbing against the use of preventive measures. The majority of well-bred women feel wounded if they believe themselves to be regarded as a means of enjoyment, not as individuals, as persons with inalienable rights. For the man also there is danger, for it is easy for him to acquire a dislike to the wife who, even though on his own initiative, occupies herself with the technique of the sexual life in a manner which he feels instinctively to be opposed to the chastity and pure mindedness demanded by every man from his wife. Ribbing, therefore, advises a certain measure of sexual abstinence in married life.

Eulenburg regards the modern diffusion and the continuous increase in the use of preventive measures as sign of decadence. Eulenburg also declares that coitus interruptus is already a frequent cause of sexual neurasthenia in women, and that its evil influence in this respect is becoming more and more frequently manifested.

The evil effects of both contraception and coitus interruptus are entirely due to the loss of seminal fluid by the parties concerned, either during or after the act, not to any assumed lack of gratification, or a failure to experience an orgasm, on the part of the female, which is proven by the fact that these practices are even more harmful to the man than they are to the woman.

Bebel (another leading gynecologist) is a declared opponent of Malthusianism.

Von Hosslin believes it to indisputable that preventive methods of sexual intercourse may cause nervous troubles, and more particularly neurasthenic disorders, manifesting themselves chiefly in the sphere of the reproductive organs.

Heart trouble may result from birth control practices. Under the title, "Cardiac Troubles due to Sexual Intercourse", **Dr. Kisch** writes:

"Among the troubles from which woman at times suffers as a result of sexual intercourse, certain cardiac disorders are especially worthy of attention. Every act of sexual intercourse in a young and sensitive woman exercises an exciting influence on the nervous mechanism controlling the cardiac movements, and this influence is more clearly manifested in a degree directly proportional to the intensity of the sexual orgasm. Similar results ensue when there is a summation of stimuli owing to excessive sexual intercourse, or contrarywise when the act of intercourse is broken off just before its physiological climax".

According to Dr. Kisch, the following diseases of the female reproductive organs result from preventive methods of sexual intercourse: chronic metritis, relaxation, retroflexion and anteflexion of the uterus, catarrhal disease of the genital mucous membrane, erosions and follicular ulceration of the portio vaginalis, oophoritis and perimetritis.

Krafft Ebing believes that "coitus interruptus, and unphysiological modes of sexual intercourse in general, are extremely potent causes of sexual neurasthenia, as potent as masturbation". Contraception and other forms of birth control are really double masturbation. They lead to more serious consequences than solitary masturbation for the following reasons:

1- *They are not inhibited by a sense of shame but are encouraged and even recommended by authorities.*

2- *There is a greater loss of seminal fluid because the act is more excessively prolonged; one's sexual organs are not only misused for the gratification of one's perverse desires, but also those of another.*

The practice of birth control results in the following diseases of the female reproductive organs: elongation of the cervix uteri (according to **Goodell**), ulceration of the cervix, infarction of the uterus and hysterical paroxysm (according to **Mensinga**), chronic hyperemia of the uterus (according to **Graffe**), perimetritis (according to **Elischer**), chronic metritis (according to **Ascher** and **Valenta**), uterine carcinoma (according to **Neugebauer** and **Pigeolot**), and premature menopause and atrophy of the uterus (according to **Lier**).

The following response was made to a questionnaire on the subject of birth control sent to a representative body of physicians:

"**Are contraceptive methods used by majority of educated married women**?" The answer to this question was "yes", invariably.

"**Are contraceptive methods capable of causing serious injury to the female genitive tract**?" The answer to this question was 75% affirmative and 25% negative.

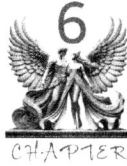

A HYGIENIC AND NATURAL METHOD OF BIRTH CONTROL

AS PROSTITUTION LED TO VENEREAL DISEASES, so contraception and other artificial methods of birth control are leading to **neurasthenia** and **cancer of the womb**. Birth control has made prostitution an almost universal practice, in and out of marriage. Mr. Thurston says: "I am impelled to the following conclusion:

1- That Nature never intended a woman to be bound to a man for life, to be compelled to occupy the same bed of habitation with him, night after night, in pregnancy and out, in order to earn her board and lodging, and to exercise her natural right to bear children.

1- That the daily and nightly juxtaposition to the male and female, which is a result of present marriage laws and customs, leads to unrestraint sexual intercourse, which perverts the natural instinct of both male and female, and makes partial prostitutes of 90% of all married women. This condition arises from the fact that married women have been led to believe that such prostitution of themselves is right and natural because it is legal, and that is necessary in order to retain the affections of their husbands.

Continual, unrestrained sexual intercourse causes the woman to become highly nervous, prematurely aged, diseased, irritable, restless, discontented, and incapable of properly caring for such children as she may bear. Among the poorer classes it leads to the propagation of many children who are not wanted, and who cannot be cared for properly when they arrive. Neglect of the children leads to disease, and makes sex perverts, degenerates and criminals.

While we maintain that contraception, as well as all other artificial methods of birth control, is unscientific, unhygienic and injurious, both to the individual and to the race. We are not in favor of uncontrolled and promiscuous breeding, nor of the conception and birth of unwanted children. We agree with the Birth Controller that the qualitative improvement of humanity is far more important than its quantitative multiplication, and that a few superior human types are much preferable to a multitude of inferior ones. But we disagree as to methods. We maintain that a more healthful, certain and scientific method of birth control exists.

Among preventative methods which require no artificial devices, one has been proposed based upon the fact that the womb is ordinarily barren from the seventeenth 'till the twenty-second day following the commencement of each menstrual flow. However, this method is unreliable, for it has been proven that spermatozoa may live for six to ten days after they are deposited, and that conception may occur on any day of the intermenstrual period. The most scientific method of birth control consists in first giving the intestinal tract a thorough cleansing through a natural diet composed of raw vegetables, fruits and nuts. Most sex desire is not natural but is due to unhealthful and stimulating foods and drinks. This is very evident in the case of alcohol, it is also so in the case of meat.

The early Christians (the Essenes), who led chaste lives, were forbidden the use of wine and animal foods. Tolstoi, who was opposed to artificial methods of birth control, as was Malthus, claimed that the natural method, namely continence, would be possible if people would use no alcohol or meat, eat with great moderation, and not be afraid of hard work. Dr. Kisch advises unmarried women who desire to reduce excessive sexual desire, to abstain from alcohol, meat and other stimulating foods. Vegetarians are generally more continent than meat eaters. Pythagoras, Plato, Aristotle, Jesus, John the Baptist, Apollonius of Tyana, St. Catherine of Siena and Leonardo da Vinci were vegetarians who led strictly chaste lives. The vegetarian diet does not reduce erotic desire by any weakening effect; rather, it gives one increased vitality, and removes irritating toxins from the blood, which have been arousing morbid sexual craving by their action upon the internal sex organ.

The gynecologist, Bebel, who is absolutely against artificial birth control, claims that desired results may be obtained in a much more healthful way by regulating the diet. He refers to the example of bees, which by a change of nutrition, can produce a new queen-bee at will. He says: "There can be no doubt whatever that the mode of nutrition has an influence on the composition of the male semen, and also on the susceptibility to the fertilization of the female ovum, hence the increase in population must, to a very important extent depend on the mode of nutrition.

If this could be definitely established, we should have in the supply of nutriment, a means of regulating the population. One has only to try the experiment of changing from a meat diet to a vegetarian one to notice a great transformation in the character of the sexual impulse. This purification of the blood brings the reproductive organs from a prolapsed, overheated, morbidly irritable condition to a healthful and firm state, as they are among animals.

The removal of an internal pressure upon the seminal vesicles (or the uterus) produced by a distended colon filled with rotting feces (as results from a meat diet), does away with the pathological centralization of erotic feeling in the genital region (an abnormality which is almost universal), thus preventing erections, which only occur in an unhealthy organism. The sex-impulse, which was previously perverted by chronic ill-health, now becomes healthy and normal. Then it finds no need for the use of artificial methods of birth control. To the healthy sexual instinct, these are disgusting.

The female genital organs, after the attainment of maturity, cannot be healthy unless they are fulfilling their natural function, reproduction. If this impulse is repressed, as occurs when birth control methods are used, the female organs become chronically irritated and inflated. The persistent urge for reproduction finds expression in a regressed form as the desire for sexual intercourse. The reproductive impulse is the driving force behind a woman's existence. When this becomes perverted, she becomes a fiend. Euripides said: "There is nothing worse than a bad woman, and nothing better than a good one".

When the possibility of reproduction is thwarted, the sexual act, to the female, becomes a narcotic, by which she can temporarily relieve the morbid irritability from which she suffers to the detriment of both herself and the male. He who made her his sexual slave, now suffers the consequences, he becomes the victim of a vampire who sucks out his life blood. There is one remedy for this condition; the adoption of a natural diet and the fulfillment of the reproductive impulse.

The male and the female are physiologically and psychologically complimentary; organs, nerve centers, and ductless glands which are most active in one, are passive in the other. Each function in a different nervous system (the male, in the central, and the female in the sympathetic). The human body is surrounded by a field of electro-magnetism, generated by electrical currents in the nerves, the radiation of the central nervous system of the male being positive and electrical in character, and those of the sympathetic nervous system of the female being negative and magnetic. The attraction between the sexes is due to an unconscious urge to unite these complementary electromagnetic radiations.

This union of soul magnetism, which may occur without physical contact (as during social dancing) is the source of joy, inspiration and invigoration resulting from the chaste association of the sexes. However, this must be differentiated from the sensations of morbid pleasure accompanying seminal emissions (the orgasm during intercourse). The former is rejuvenating and life giving; the latter is deadening and devitalizing. The one is healthy, the other is pathological.

The belief that the insertion of the penis into the vagina, followed by onanistic friction and by the discharge of seminal fluid is divinely ordained as the only normal fulfillment of the sex impulse (a falsity which has been impressed upon us during early childhood by the bad example of our parents, and by the instructions we have received from companions of the street and school) is a superstition which has wrought havoc with mankind. No healthy, undomesticated animal engages in such perverse activity (for, all will be shown later, the reproductive act, among healthy animals, is of a very different nature).

Contraception, contrary to the opinions of would be eugenists, leads to an inferior race. Such knowledge is more accessible to the educated than to the illiterate classes. Also all who thus misuse their reproductive organs become incapable of ever giving birth to normal children. Their future progeny, if they have any, will be diseased and feeble-minded (unless they revitalize themselves, previous to conception, by hygienic and continent living). Contraceptive addicts destroy their own, as well as their future children's health. While in the animal, sex has only one expression, procreation, in man it has another, a psychological and social one. The great error of the human race has been to seek the fulfillment of the latter purpose through means designed for the accomplishment of the former.

The sex organs have two normal functions: reproduction and internal secretion. A healthy organism will use them in no other way. An unhealthy one, however, whose sex organs are irritated by toxins in the blood (produced by alcohol, meat or tobacco), will seek to remove this irritation by friction, followed by a seminal discharge. Such an act, whether the hand or the organ of the opposite sex is used for the purpose, is masturbation pure and simple. Sexual intercourse is therefore a vicarious form of masturbation. One who acquires true physiological health through a natural diet has no such perverse desires.

Every natural impulse is good, for it has an organic function to perform. It is only the perversion of the natural impulse which is evil. The original function of the sense of taste, which was to select physiologically beneficial nutriment, has in most people been lost. The tongue has been made into an organ of pleasure, to the detriment of the organism. In a similar manner the reproductive instinct has been perverted. And it was the perversion of the nutritive instinct (as is evident by the domestication and artificial feeding of animals) that led to the perversion of the sexual instinct. Therefore, by regaining our natural nutritive instinct, we will thereby regain our natural sexual instinct. Since the sex relationship is a blending of magnetism, there is no reason why the reproductive organs need have any part of it. Magnetic vitality is not centered in the pelvic region but pervades the entire organism, being especially strong around the head.

A hygienic diet will remove the internal irritation which causes a desire to masturbate while in soul-union with one we love. This is the only healthy and natural method of birth control. Vegetarians desire no other one. Since it involves a conservation of vital fluid by both parties, it is rejuvenating, healing and strengthening, instead of devitalizing. However, this magnetic relationship should not be engaged in too frequently or promiscuously. It should not be indulged in during the year previous to conception.

It is only recommended to those who might otherwise destroy themselves by more harmful practices, even as dairy products are recommended to those who are changing from a meat to a vegetarian diet. The sex organs have two normal functions: procreation and internal secretions. Any other use of them is a perversion which must lead to pathological consequences. This is the opinion of the great gynecologist, Hegar, who says:

"Gratification on the sexual impulse, gives rise in women to the formation and growth of tumors, cause numerous mechanical disturbances, and opens the way to infection. The numerous and various disasters which are

brought upon the world by unbridled and unregulated sexual passion can be prevented only by enlightenment, moderation and continence".

Magnetic interchange, in which the reproductive organs have no part (in which no masturbation occurs) is the most rational method of birth control. Those who imagine that such a sex life is too idealistic or Platonic for them have only to stop drinking and smoking, and to cleanse their digestive tract through a vegetarian diet, to find out that it is not, that instead, it is the only healthy and natural expression of the sex impulse, of which the other is a pathological perversion. Localization of erotic feeling in the genital region is due to the irritation and stimulation produces by meat, fish, eggs, coffee, tea, alcohol and tobacco.

When the blood is purified, such morbid sensations and desires cease. The reproductive organs are then used only for their natural purpose which is 'procreation'. The chaste happiness attending the blending of soul-magnetism replaces the perverse pleasure of seminal emissions. Those who substitute this chaste sexual relationship for the old, devitalizing, pathogenic sexual intercourse' will discover its great superiority. One leads to increased health; while the other leads to disease. One results in happiness, peace and satisfaction, the other produces only a morbid irritability, a pathological craving which increases with its gratification. One leads to longevity, the other leads to premature senility and death. One recharges, heals and rejuvenates the body; the other weakens and destroys it. One makes marriage a perpetual courtship, the other to degeneracy.

Commentary by **LIQUID METAL**

I'm pretty sure that when Dr. Bernard mentions the word "vegetarian", he means "vegan" as we use it in our time. The word itself tells that it's about vegetation (fruit and vegetables). So no animal products (milk, eggs, yogurt etc.) Try to not be swayed away or distracted from erotic or any sexual content. Not only that the content itself will keep your sexual energy localized in your genital area, but it will also keep the overall energy stuck or concentrated in the lower chakras or energy centers. Your kundalini will not rise up the spine if its path is blocked from stagnant energy.

PART III

The Laws of
Dietetics

"Behold, I have given you every herb bearing seed, which is upon the face of all earth, and every tree, in which is the fruit of a tree yielding seed. To you shall be for meat. And to every beast of the earth, and to every fowl of the air, and to everything that creepeth upon the earth, wherein there is life, I have given every green herb for meat" – Genesis I

"There is no disease, bodily or mental, which adoption of vegetable diet and pure water has not infallibly mitigated" – Percy B Shelly, A Vindication of the Natural Diet

VEGETARIANISM - THE FOUNDATION OF RACE GENERATION

VEGETARIANISM HAS BEEN CHIEFLY CONSIDERED BY MOST WRITERS on the subject in relation to its hygienic and health value. However, it has an important significance in relation to eugenics, the science of race regeneration. It is not without reason that the mothers of past supermen, the founders of the world's religions, as Chrishna, founder of Brahmanism, Gautama, founder of Buddhism etc., were raised on a vegetarian diet, as were the mothers of Samuel, Samson and the Christian Savior.

Concerning Devaki, the virgin mother of Chrishna, it was said, "No animal food ever touched his lips". This reminds one of the characters of Mary, the Mother of Jesus, as given in the 'Gospel of Mary', where it is said that no animal food ever touched her lips. Maia, Buddha's mother, was supposed to have always lived in obedience to the *"five great commandments"*. One of these states: "Thou shalt abstain from destroying or causing the destruction of any living thing (which means a vegetarian diet)"; and another, "Thou shalt abstain from the use of intoxicants". Previous to Samson's conception, an angel gave his mother the following command: "Thou shalt conceive and bear a son. Now therefore beware, I pray you, and drink not wine nor strong drink, and eat not unclean thing (meat)".

St. David of Wales was born from a mother who, during gestation led a most faithful life, for from that time of conception she lived on bread and water only. The mother of Honen Shonin, a Chinese Buddhist saint, during the whole period of pregnancy was free from pain. She strictly abstained from wine, meat and the five prohibited vegetables.

The following illustrious figures in history were advocates of vegetarianism: Zoroaster, Moses, Isaiah, Daniel, Buddha, Pythagoras, Empedocles, Hesiod, Ovid, Socrates, Plato, Aristotle, Dyogenes the Cynic, Zeno the Stoic, Plautus, Quintus, Sextus, Seneca, Apollonius of Tyana, Porphyry, Proclus, Plutarch, Petrarch, St. Catherine of Siena, Leonardo da Vinci, Rousseau, Voltaire, Shelley, Pope, Wesley, Franklin, Linnaeus, Thoreau, Richard Wagner, Tolstoi, and Maeterlinck. The Pythagoreans, the Essenes (the early Christians), and the followers of St. Francis, St. Theresa and Tolstoi were vegetarians. The Jesus and John the Baptist of the Gospels, since they were Essenes, were both vegetarians. Vegetarianism was one of the teachings of the Christian Savior which the carnivorous founders of the church suppressed.

Not only the intellectually, but also the physically most superior types of humanity were vegetarians. Adam Smith, in his "Wealth of Nations" says: "The brave Spartans who, for muscular power, physical energy and ability to endure hardship, perhaps stand unequalled in the history of nations, were vegetarians. The departure from their simple diet was soon followed by their decline. The armies of Greece and Rome, in the times of their unparalleled conquests, subsisted on vegetable productions.

In the training for the public games in Greece, where muscular strength was to be exhibited in all its various forms, vegetable food was adhere to; nut when flesh meat was adopted afterwards, those hitherto athletic men became sluggish and stupid. From two-thirds to three-fourths of the whole human family, from the creation of the species to the present time, have subsisted entirely, or nearly so, on vegetable food; and always, when their alimentary supplies of this kind have been abundant and of good quality, and their habits have been in other respects correct, they have been well nourished and well sustained in all the physiological interests of their nature".

WHY ANIMAL FOODS ARE UNHYGIENIC

Meat is an unnecessary, toxic, pathogenic and exceedingly injurious article of food. This is so because of the poisonous waste products which exist in all animal tissue, particularly after death. For several hours after it is killed, the cells of the animal's body continue to live, absorbing oxygen and food material form, and returning carbonic dioxide and toxic substances to the blood.

The excretions of these waste products, through the ordinary channels, is then no longer possible; these remain in the venous blood that saturates the flesh. It is these toxic excreta in meat (chemically identical with, and having the same odor as urine) which are dissolved in beef tea and broth, and which give it its characteristic taste. When they are washed away, leaving only the protein fibers of the flesh (which is the only possible nourishment in meat), this food is tasteless. It is, therefore, these toxins which the meat-eater craves, when they are absent, meat loses its charms.

Meat is heart-stimulant; the poisonous toxins which it contains act directly upon the heart. This is demonstrated by the fact that the average heartbeats of a vegetarian are 58 to the minute, while those of meat-eaters are 72. Fifteen hundred extra heart strokes every twenty-four hours result in a very appreciable strain upon the vital forces. Meat eating thus causes high blood pressure, heart disease, hardening of the arteries and premature senility.

It is a physiological fact that the intestines of man, like those of other frugivorous animals, are for times the length of the intestine of carnivorous animals. Those of the latter, besides being short, have a smooth interior lining, to insure the rapid passage and assimilation of their putrescible contents. The human intestines, on the other hand, are convoluted, as are those of animals which live on vegetable foods.

When meat is put into the long human intestines, which are designed for the slow digestion of frugivorous nutriment, it quickly ferments and decays, generating poisonous toxins which are carried by the blood throughout the body, leading to a great number of diseases. While the blood of the carnivorous animal is practically free from uric acid, that of the carnivorous man is invariably saturated with it. Uric acid causes rheumatism, gout and kidney diseases.

That meat is not a natural food for man is shown by the fact that the instinctive pleasure with which the animal kills its prey is normally foreign to his nature; as also is that derived from eating warm, raw flesh, dripping with blood. Meat generally has to be cooked, salted and seasoned in order to disguise its origin. After observing the slaughter of an animal, one loses one's appetite to eat it. It is only because economical conditions force certain individuals to spend their lives on such brutalizing work that others eat as much meat as they do.

The craving for meat is not due to its nourishing, but to its stimulating properties. Meat, like alcohol, is in a state of bacterial fermentation. This decay, though it may be inhibited by cold storage or chemicals, proceeds at an accelerated rate as soon as it enters the warm intestines. The toxins thus generated, by their stimulating effects upon the heart, create the illusion that meat gives strength.

Meat not only has a similar physiological effect as has alcohol, but, as Maeterlinck, in his "Buried Temple", points out, it causes a desire for alcohol. A mild stimulant, frequently repeated, loses its effect, and a stronger one is sought. Meat-eating thus leads to smoking, drinking, drug-addiction and sex perversion. As a result of its irritating effect upon the genital organs, meat leads to masturbation among children and sex excess among adults.

What has been said about meat equally applies to fowl, fish and eggs, all of which are unnatural and unhealthy foods. Chicken and eggs are powerful sex-stimulants, particularly when eaten by children— for the hen's life is continuously absorbed in sex activity, and the egg is an ovarian product. The word "fowl" is phonetically correct (foul), for the chicken is a filthy creature which feeds on worms, grasshoppers, flies and other insects. Eggs, no matter in what way they are prepared, are extremely indigestible.

Milk, after the period of weaning, is an unnecessary and unnatural food. Cow's milk is chemically unfit for human consumption. The large curds which it forms are unable to pass through the delicate intestinal wall, upon which they deposit as a greasy, adhesive coating which interferes with digestion. Cream, because of its higher concentration of large fat globules, is still more constipating. Butter is an overconcentrated fat which does not form healthy tissue. Instead, it oozes out from the skin, yielding a perceptible odor. Fermented cheese, since they are in a state of bacterial decay, are, like meat, very injurious.

The PROTEIN REQUIREMENT

The average individual eats far more protein than has been found to be physiologically necessary. This excessive protein causes a strain upon the heart and kidneys. While extra quantities of carbohydrates may be stored as fat, the waste products of protein, beyond that which the kidneys are able to eliminate, remain in the blood as acid toxins which poison the tissues of the body.

According to recent experiments, the protein requirement has previously been placed three times too high. It has been estimated that the average individual normally requires no more than half an ounce to an ounce and a half of protein each day. Physiological experimenters of the past, after measuring the end-products of protein decomposition daily excreted, have wrongly supposed that these were derived from the disintegration of muscular tissues; and that an equivalent amount of protein had to be present in the diet. But the fact was not considered that this elimination of protein and products takes place whether there is muscular activity or not, and that it is dependent upon the quantity of protein eaten and the concentration of its acid toxins in the blood. If less protein is used, less elimination of its end-products occurs.

A sufficiently high concentration of alkaline elements in the blood prevents the premature cleavage and disintegration of the protein molecule, and thus reduces the protein requirement. **Protein does not supply muscular energy**; all it contains is building materials with which to construct new tissues. As the child grows older, it requires less and less protein; at maturity, a minimum amount is needed. This is shown by the gradual diminution in the protein-content of mother's milk during lactation.

Seeds *(sesame, sunflower, pumpkin, pine kernels, etc.)* *are the best substitutes for animal proteins*. They contain on the average, several times more protein than meat, which has only 15-20 per cent. The protein of seeds, besides being more digestible and less putrescible than that of meat, not forming acid toxins as does the latter, is balanced by carbohydrates, fats, minerals and vitamins, all of which are absent from cooked meat.

The humble peanut contains 29% protein, 61% fat and 11% carbohydrates, while beef only has 18% protein, 5% fat and no carbohydrates; and eggs, 12% protein, 12% fat and 5% carbohydrates. Nut-butters, made from raw peanuts, almonds or coconuts, are cheaper and more nutritious than cow's butter. Legumes (which contain from 20 to 25% protein) may also be used as substitutes for meat, fowl, fish and eggs.

WHY MAN'S NATURAL DIET IS FRUGIVOROUS

Animals may be classified, according to their dietetic habits, into four major groups;

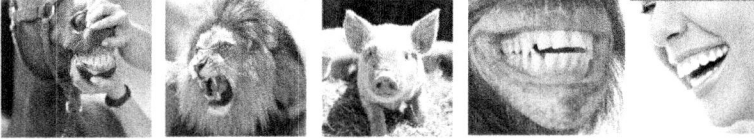

Herbivorous (the horse)
Carnivorous (the lion)
Omnivorous (the pig)
Frugivorous (the ape)

As is evident from a consideration of the following anatomical facts, man is a frugivorous creature; his natural diet consists of fruits and nuts. This is so for the following reasons:

1- Herbivorous and omnivorous animals have hoofs in order to roam around on grassy plains, carnivorous ones have claws to grasp their prey, while frugivorous ones have hands, to pick fruit from the trees.

2- Carnivorous animals drink by lapping up water with their tongue, while man and herbivorous animals drink by suction. The tongue of the former is rough, that of the latter is smooth.

3- Carnivorous animals sleep by day, men and herbivorous ones sleep by night.

4- The teeth of carnivorous animals have five times the hardness of the teeth of man and frugivorous animals. The former have slightly developed incisors and pointed molars, while the latter have well developed incisors and blunt molars, The argument that man is naturally carnivorous, or omnivorous, because of his "canine" teeth is fallacious, for these eye-teeth are much longer in the frugivorous ape which uses them to crack nuts.

5- According to Huxley's classification of animals, by the type of placenta, man is frugivorous. The placenta of the carnivorous animal is of the zonary type; that of omnivorous and herbivorous animals is of the non-deciduate type; while that of man and frugivorous animals is of the discoidal type.

6- While all other animals are four-footed, the higher ape and man have two hands and two feet, with flat nails instead of claws or hoofs. The former look from side to side as they crawl, the latter look straight ahead as they walk. The former have tails and mammary glands on the abdomen, the latter are without tails, and have mammary glands only on the breasts.

7- The alimentary canal of the carnivorous animal is three times the length of its trunk, it is smooth and non-sacculated so that its putrescible contents may be quickly assimilated and eliminated. That of the ape and man, however, is twelve times the length of the trunk, being lined with sacculated valvular folds, so that its frugivorous contents may be retained for a relatively longer period.

8- The stomach of carnivorous animals is a simple sac, that of herbivorous animals has three or four compartments; while that of frugivorous ones has a duodenum, or a small second stomach.

9- The appendix of carnivorous animals is very small, that of herbivorous animals is larger, that of frugivorous ones is still larger, and that of man is largest of all.

10- Carnivorous animals have atrophied sweat glands and have no pores on the skin, Herbivorous and frugivorous animals do have pores and functional sweat glands.

11- The salivary glands of carnivorous animals are very small and produce acid secretion which has little effect upon starch, those of man and frugivorous animals on the other hand, are well developed, and produce an alkaline secretion which does affect starch.

12- The gastric juice of carnivorous animals has a decomposing and antiseptic influence upon meat, while that of man is far too weak to disintegrate its tough fibers.

13- The liver of carnivorous animals is very much larger than that of man and frugivorous animals, and is able to destroy proportionately ten to fifteen times as much uric acid.

Commentary by LIQUID METAL

It is custom in our modern society to accompany lunch or dinner with different kinds of green salads. If you just have meat, it ferments, now if you consume also salads, which should take much less time to be digested, the salad or any vegetable or fruit that is consumed within two hours of having consumed meat, it will also ferment. Our system is designed so that what we eat passes out after it's maximum digestion time is reached.

Even if you eat fruit or vegetables after you ate pizza or pasta, the same logic/fact applies. Except fruit, vegetables, herbs, seeds and nuts, anything else is dead food. As a matter of fact, it should not be called food. I have fallen many times in the trap of my own thinking, or in the trap of my taste buds or stomach hunger. Don't let flavor and hunger control your higher faculty.

Some information written in this book is about meat eating, vegetarian diet, parthenogenesis etc. It might not be understood and then practiced by anyone who doesn't believe that people can live for hundreds of years if a strict vegetarian diet and continence (full chaste) life is followed. If you think that living to a 100 years of age is something to be proud of, then you deny the potential of your whole being and what you are designed for. Everyone can learn from their own mistakes; intelligent is someone who learned from other people's mistakes. Real food is that which doesn't require to be seasoned. Real food is eaten raw in its natural state such as fruit and vegetables.

Disease will first whisper at you before it talks, if you continue to ignore it, it will then scream, but by that time, it might be too late. Every time a friend or a kin gets sick or dies, it empowers me more than before to take better care of my health. Life, or the Universe will let you know what to do through different circumstances, through your friends, siblings, random strangers etc. Pay attention to synchronicities. Anything in life, or anyone in your life who tries to hurt or to help/heal you, is there to teach you lessons.

You don't have to eat every time you are hungry. Your body produces two hormones, Leptin and Ghrelin, one is the hormone that tells you that you are hungry, while the other tells you that you are full. Most people eat when they should not eat, and they don't eat when they should eat. This is because those two hormones are over stimulated from processed/toxic foods and drinks and they give false alarm.

Little curiosity, "**carnivorous**" is an anagram for "**coronavirus**". "**Veganism**" is an anagram for "**saving me**". Is it a coincidence? I don't think so.

You read the difference of our physiological body compared to the carnivorous animals (the 13 points). Even after reading those anatomical facts, if you still think that man is naturally carnivorous, then good for you. Nobody can help you beside yourself, no matter how many facts you are presented with.

I often hear people say that vegetables are alive and that they have pain when we eat them. Of course this derives from false information they read online or in some books. If we go by that logic, then we should not breathe either since air is alive. Everything is alive, even a rock's atoms are vibrating 24/7; although we don't see a rock moving by itself. We have hands to grab the food that doesn't escape from us. No animal would willingly want to be slaughtered. What if I tell you that originally, even animals would not eat other animals, would you believe me?

That some animals eat other animals, happens because throughout time, our way of life, our psyche has poisoned the animal's world (electromagnetism or consciousness). If you were to raise a baby lion and a bunny or a lamb in the same house/farm, then you would cause the lion reconnect with true nature of life. Of course, the lion may still eat another animal if it's the first generation. But if the same lion procreates in the same environment a couple or more generations, then the offsprings would not have the urge or the drive to hunt or eat another animal. Applies the same for people. You can disagree if you wish.

If the government decided to push the eating of the cats and dogs in the western world, after a couple of generations, people will be eating cats and dogs. So, why is it okay to eat chicken, pigs, cows but not cats and dogs? You don't need anyone to tell you what's moral. Look within the depth of your true being and you will know the true answer if it's okay to slaughter/eat another sentient being or not.

Also, all meats, with no exception, have parasites in them. The parasites will cause you to become horny, especially when you are on a path to cleansing your physical vessel. The parasites, just like anything alive, have consciousness therefore, the parasites aim to transfer themselves to a new host. Even just a simple kiss will transfer some of your parasites onto another person and vice versa.

Be mindful of whom you let inside your temple.

If you go full vegan, which means raw food only, food that is grown in and on the ground, I advise you to not neglect all forms of nuts such as, walnuts, hazelnuts, brazil nuts etc. so that you get supplied with good/healthy fats that your body needs. What you eat is very crucial also to the mineral deficiency or Cell Salt that everyone is deficient of, based on each individual's zodiacal sign. For example, if you are Gemini, you are deficient of the Cell Salt "Potassium Chloride. Hazelnut is one of the foods someone born under the Gemini Zodiacal sign that should consume on a regular basis. For more on the cell salts subject, check books by George W. Carey. Also, check out these two books about the same subject:

To Be Reborn by Tamo A. Replica

The Science Of The Sacred Secretion by Victoria Loalow

Since I began consuming only fruit, vegetable seeds and nuts these are some changes that I noticed:

1- *I have been dreaming nonstop at night, beautiful and sometimes random dreams that don't make sense and yet, they will make sense when the time is right.*

2- *I don't even need to nap anymore. Before going on a raw diet, I felt like I needed to nap every day and I was napping most of the days. If after lunch or dinner you feel sleepy/tired, either you are consuming the wrong food or you are eating too much. Eating should make us feel energized and not tired.*

3- *I barely urinate anymore. When you consume toxic food and drinks, it causes the body to want to expel the toxins, and water is needed to expel any toxins or foreign organisms. Since I severely changed my diet, my system has been balanced and it uses the right amount of water needed to function. There is still more work to do in improving our health, no matter how healthy we eat.*

4- *My urine is only clear/white daily, rarely any shades of yellow or light brown, and barely any red color when I consume beet juice from raw beet roots as opposed to previous lifestyle where the urine from beet juice would be red like blood.*

5- *I have time for everything. Ample time to spend. Just by not needing to nap, I gain 2-3 hours more per day, plus being clear minded,* *makes me efficient with time. Before, I was not balanced emotionally or mentally, therefore, one makes mistakes and unnecessarily wastes time.*

6- Coffee and tea, especially coffee causes you to have to urinate earlier than you should, which means that the body in the process of trying to expel the toxins from the coffee (coffee is a neurotoxin, meaning it is a foreign organism to the body), will expel or leech stem cells, nutrients, minerals/cell salt, monoatomic gold etc. out of your body through urine. All these beneficial nutrients, stem cells etc., mentioned above, when leeched out, cause your body to weaken. Not only that, but your cells will also dehydrate. Cell dehydration means premature aging and early death. I have never felt as strong as I feel now on a raw food diet.

7- My eyes' color changed. A while back, I read online that when you are on a raw fruit and vegetable diet, your eye color changes. I dismissed it at that time, I didn't believe it. But how could you believe something that you don't know. We shouldn't believe anything anyway, unless we verify it through personal experiences. As always, we should keep an open mind that what we don't know may be true. I was driving somewhere and checked the mirror for a second and to my amazement I looked at my eyes' color change. Throughout my life, up to a month ago, my eyes were hazel color. Now half of the outside perimeter of my irises is light blue, while the inner half of the perimeter is light brown. No one in my family ever had blue eyes, and definitely none of them were on a raw food diet either. The lesson I got from this is to not ridicule or deny information that I don't know or that I don't believe it to be true.

8- My dark hair color is returning. I had a lot of grey hair. I am not old, I do not feel old at all because I don't believe in aging, nor dying, but I am fairly certain that by wasting too much seminal emissions throughout the last 2 decades (until a few years ago) is what caused it. Food has played a small part too; I usually consumed decent and healthy food. But now, since I have been on a full raw food diet, I have seen many changes.

Many people don't do anything to fix their health until it is too late. Disease, first winks at you, then it will whisper, and finally it will scream. By then, it will be too late, you may still reverse something, as in adding a few more years to your life, but forget reaching a 100 years of age, let alone living for hundreds of years. May I remind you that to add decades and centuries to your life span, eating raw fruit, vegetables, seeds and nuts is not enough. Chastity is equally important.

I just remembered, once, there was a man who was a virgin at that time. After a bit of talk, I told him "Man, you don't know what you are losing by not having sex". Of course at that time I was consumed by lust. He told me "Man, you don't know what you are losing by not consuming heroin". He never consumed heroin, he said that to get me to understand that you cannot lose something you didn't have it in the first place. But it took me years to truly understand what he meant. Be careful of your attachments to lust, people, ideologies and certain foods and drinks.

"Attachments are the poisons that dig your grave one shovel at a time" – Liquid Metal

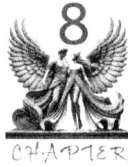

EVIL OF BREAD ADDICTION – WHY WHEAT IS AN UNNATURAL FOOD

GRAINS (EXCEPT CORN) ARE NOT PROVIDED by nature in a form for man to eat; they are not natural foods. Starch, which is their main constituent, must be transformed into fruit sugar, through the action of many different enzymes, before it may be assimilated. Therefore, it is a great saving of vital energy to obtain this fruit sugar directly from sweet fruit, such as grapes. Grain in all forms should be eliminated from the diet and replaced by the predigested carbohydrates of fruits. These are obtained in their natural state, balanced by organic minerals and vitamins (which counterbalance their acidic forming tendency), while the starch of grain, which is tasteless and indigestible when eaten raw, is usually cooked or baked, after which its vitamins are destroyed and its minerals are inorganic and unassimilable.

Whole wheat bread, therefore, contains absolutely no organic mineral or vitamins. The starch of nuts is more digestible than that of grain. Those who feed horses are very careful never to give them grain unless they are doing heavy work; otherwise there is danger of the horse getting sick. Yet the horse, which is herbivorous animal, is much better able to digest grain than can the human being. A horse fed on grain ages sooner than one fed on grass. The Argentinian Gauchos, who subsist on a diet practically free from grain, live to the average age of 125 years. Herodotus relates that a Persian ambassador, when asked by the Ethiopians how long his people lived, answered, "70 years". The latter accounted for their short lives because of the fact that they ate "dirt" which was the word used for bread.

Bread-eating, like alcohol drinking, is a perverse habit. Both indulgences result in the hardening of the arteries. The bacterial fermentation of bread changes part of the starch into alcohol. Once inside the stomach, more of the starch, by the action of the acid gastric juices, is transformed into alcohol. Bread eating is thus a vicarious form of alcoholic indulgence.

Fermented bread is preferred by most people to the more hygienic unleavened bread because of its higher alcoholic content. Thus, the desire for bread and alcohol is the same; it is a desire for the eating of fermenting material whose toxins may stimulate the heart and the sex organ. The immediate effect of bread upon the human body (which is not noticeable when bread is habitually used, but it is very evident when it is eaten for the first time in several month) is very similar to that produced by a mild alcoholic, namely, brain stupor. This is due to the fact that bread, like alcohol, absorbs oxygen from the blood, which it saturates with carbonic acid. This leads to a precipitation of carbon in the cerebral capillaries, which obstructs the circulation of the brain. This does not occur when raw sweet corn, which is the only healthful for of grain, is eaten.

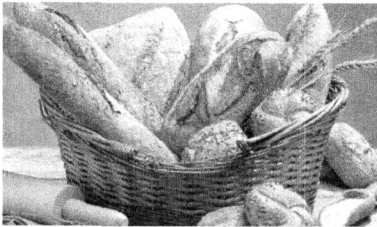

Whole wheat bread is even more acid-forming than white bread. The latter is constipating and mucus-forming, while the sharp, bristle brain of the former injuriously irritates and cuts into the delicate mucous lining of the intestines, producing a chronic diarrhea which is mistaken for a laxative action. Contrary to the opinion of dietetic novices, whole wheat bread in not "health food".

White flour products, corn starch and refined cereals (such as bolted cornmeal, pearled barley, white rice and commercial oatmeal) are very unhygienic, for their embryo and cellulose have been removed, leaving only the pasty, constipating and mucous-forming starch. By the acids which they generate in the blood, these foods these foods deprive the body of calcium (needed by the bones) and phosphorus (required by the nervous system). It is for this reason that a diet consisting largely of refined cereals causes rickets (a bone disease) and beriberi (a nervous disease), which are due not to the fact that those already in the body are dissolved, for a period of fasting will not bring on these conditions.

Dogs fed on white bread die sooner than those not fed at all. The use of white bread by children retards their normal physical and mental development. White flour has been bleached by chlorine, which is a poisonous gas. The human digestive organs were never designed for the assimilation of cereal starch. This is proven by a study of the as yet unperverted human being, the infant, who is incapable of digesting starch.

Young children instinctively avoid cooked cereals. Starch changes into alcohol; and the continued use of bread leads to a carbon deposit in the stomach. It has been demonstrated that only 5% of starch is changed into sugar by the saliva, the remainder being sent in an undigested form to the duodenum. The pancreas is then overcooked to manufacture sufficient enzymes to change this into sugar. This results in diabetes, a more severe pancreas-exhaustion than is ordinarily possessed by the average bread eater.

The various grains are degenerate and dried up variations of a primordial grain, corns. Raw sweet corn, right off the stalk, is the most hygienic form of grain. Since corn does not have the tendency to form calcareous deposits or to cause seminal emissions as have wheat and rye, it should be used as the staple grain. For those who are weaning off from the use of bread and cereals, the following tasty and nutritious unleavened corn bread may be recommended. It is made of mixing unbolted, stone-ground cornmeal (not the bolted and steel-cut kind) with water, adding olive oil and honey, and baking it in flat thin layers for about ten to fifteen minutes. This unleavened bread, eaten together with a raw vegetable salad, is an excellent cure for constipation. The fermentation of bread by yeast is a process of incipient rotting; while baking powder is an injurious chemical. Therefore, bread should always be eaten in an unleavened form.

One subject to the bread-eating habit desires this food at every meal; but when no bread is eaten for a sufficient length of time, the craving for it disappears. This shows that bread is not naturally required by the human organism, and that the desire for it is an artificial one. Carob (St. John's bread) is a sunbaked bread which Nature has provided for man to eat. It should be used instead of all other grains, including corn. While the starch of grain must be transformed by the enzymes of the saliva into maltose, and by those of the duodenum and small intestines, into dextrose, carob contains an invert sugar which is immediately transformed into dextrose and assimilated in the stomach. Grapes, however, are even superior to carob, for they contain pure dextrose, or grape sugar, in a fresh form. Grapes are the best substitutes for bread and cereals.

🖋 *Commentary by* LIQUID METAL

How does that bread image make you feel? I don't know you, but it made me like baking some bread. Which means that I am not completely free of the bread addiction. I don't eat bread anymore, but I only recently stopped consuming bread that's why when I see bread it still makes me want to eat but I won't fall for any image, smell or bread talk. It takes a gigantic will to let go of bread in my case, or anything else in other people cases, based on each individual's addiction.
Bread was the last thing I wouldn't let go. It was like a drug to me. I would eat bread with everything.

While you are reading this book, every time you feel overwhelmed or triggered as to foods you must stop eating, try to remember the title of the book. This information is about becoming a perfectly healthy being. Of course, if you are someone that are home all day, you have a much better chance at incorporating a strictly vegetarian (vegan) diet. It can be done, I am doing it, even though I have to go to work for someone else for now. I also practice continence, which is very important.

A lot of people who try to change their diet into veganism/ vegetarianism, get sick or are still not satisfied with their health, that's because they continually leak their life force (semen/ovum and other secretions). Losing your life force is much more detrimental than not eating healthily. The more we learn, the more we realize we have much more to learn.

> *"When we realize that we are ignorant, that makes us intelligent by default"*

When we think we know it all, that's when we fall behind. It is very important to be an observer of the information in this book, don't let the memories of certain tasty foods you had in your life, or certain sexual memories, or anything that gratifies your senses, blind your rational mind and divine intuition.

P.S. Dr. Bernard uses both the words "fruit" and "fruits". English is my third language, but from what I know, "fruit" is both singular and plural. Perhaps 6 decades ago they used the words fruit and fruits interchangeably.

HARMFUL CONDIMENTS, STIMULANTS AND NARCOTICS

THE INJURIOUS EFFECTS OF

Sugar

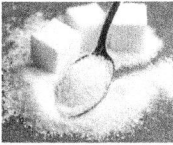

Salt

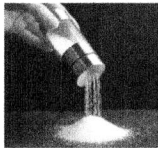

Coffee

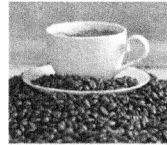

Tea

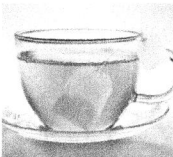

Tobacco

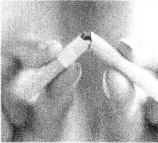

Alcohol

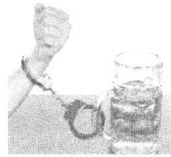

SUGAR

REFINED CANE SUGAR (white or brown), glucose, saccharine, molasses and their products such as (candy, chocolate, ice cream, soda water, fruit preserves, jelly, pie, pastry and cake) are extremely harmful. White sugar has been treated with chemicals, and has been bleached by animal bones. Because of this high temperature to which it has been heated, in the process of "refining", it has been reduced to a crystalline, inorganic state, in which it cannot be assimilated by the cells of the human body.

The candy eating habit in children is a vicarious form of alcoholism, for white sugar changes in the stomach into alcohol. This is why prohibition in the United States was followed by an increased use of confectioneries. Alcohol is fermented sugar. In eating a form of sugar which readily ferments, we take an incipient alcohol into the system.

"Although its effect upon the system is highly stimulating, the energizing power of sugar is exceeded only by its reaction of fermentation, much like an explosion, resulting in the absorption of what remains of the oxygen in the stomach. After food enters the stomach, one of two things physiologically happen, either digestion or fermentation. The common theory that sugar is both strengthening and fattening is due to the alcohol in which there is absolutely no nourishing or fattening materials. From this we unconsciously turn our gastric laboratory into an alcoholic distillery.

Sugar, when thus converted into alcohol, has the semblance of giving extraordinary strength momentarily to the individual, similar to the common effect on the system when taken in the for of spirits, or liquor, when drunk as an intoxicating beverage. But instead of strengthening and vitalizing the system, sugar, in fact, does the opposite by using the body up and breaking it down. It has a peculiar action of leeching the blood from the tissues. As it is possible for the body to utilize but a small portion of the amount of sugar actually consumed, the organs are overtaxed and have a burdensome task of eliminating and ridding themselves of the surplus.

The fruits and natural foods contain in abundance all the sugar needed to meet the requirements of the body". - Hayes, Health Educator

The physiological effects of white sugar and alcohol are almost identical. Both rapidly oxidize, absorbing oxygen from the blood and precipitating inorganic carbon on the mucous lining of the digestive tract and along the interior wall of the arteries. The heat generated by this combustion has been mistaken by physiologists for the energy-producing quality of sugar. Such heat is identical with the resulting from the drinking of alcohol. It is due to the oxidation of carbon compounds in the stomach. Carbon dioxide is thus generated; and the blood is filled with carbonic acid. This, chemically combines with the calcium of the bone and teeth, forming a calcium carbonate precipitate which leads to calcareous hardening of the arteries. It is for this reason that children who eat much candy remain small and suffer from dental decay. Often, the taking of sugar into the body is quickly followed by a toothache. The calcium in the blood regulates the beating of the heart. White sugar, by causing a precipitation of this calcium, causes the heart to beat excessively fast. Similar effects follow the use of alcohol. The heart is also forced to beat faster because of the lowered concentration of oxygen in the blood.

The effects of white sugar, like those of alcohol, are most pernicious upon the brain. The child addicted to candy experiences a mild intoxication after the indulgence. The saturation of the blood with carbonic acid interferes with the cerebral circulation, dulls the brain and retards mental development. If this is true of white sugar, is it not true of all sugars? We must differentiate between a natural and fresh sugar, such as in the grape, and an artificial and preserved sugar, such as white sugar, or even raisins.

The sugar of the grape, dextrose, immediately passes into the blood after entering the stomach. The presence of vital force within it prevents its fermentation. However, should grapes stand a few days, and should this vital force be dissipated, it will commence to ferment, or turn into alcohol.

Raw cane sugar, like grapes, is very nutritious. It does not ferment. And as the raisin in the grape whose fermentation has been prevented by being dehydrated, so white sugar is a dehydrated and crystallized form of cane sugar. When such preserved sugar is eaten, moister is suddenly added to it. This leads to an outbursts of its inhibited fermentation, especially in the presence of the hydrochloric acid of the stomach. Therefore, dried fruits, such as prunes, figs, dates, apricots, peaches and raisins, though far more healthful than white sugar, are not truly hygienic foods. Besides, as usually obtained, they have been treated with sulphur, or artificially sweetened.

As substitutes for white sugar, honey, maple sugar and carob sugar (pulverized St. John's bread, which contains 55% natural invert sugar and 25% protein) may be recommended. None of these, however, are as hygienic as the fresh dextrose of grapes. Saccharine (a coal-tar product), glucose (which has been treated with chemicals) and molasses (which contains poisonous sulphur dioxide), the three chief constituents of children's candies, are all very injurious.

SALT

Table salt is an inorganic chemical; it has never been transformed by the vital process of the plant. It acts upon the body as a drug rather than as food, seriously injuring the digestive organs, heart and kidneys. It rapidly absorbs moisture, and dries up waste matter which should otherwise be eliminated. In this way, it causes obesity. Salt addiction results in high blood pressure. Celery salt (pulverized dehydrated celery) is a hygienic and organic form of sodium chloride. This is now on the market; and it should be substituted for common salt.

"To be sure, we need common salt, just as we need iron and potash, and sulfur and lime, and other mineral salts; but no one thinks of sprinkling lime and potash and iron filings over his food, just the same. There is no more reason why we should sprinkle sodium chloride, or common salt, over our food, than there is why we should sprinkle any of the other salts. Both are equally mineral substances; and hence both are equally unusable by the system. Salt can have no more effect upon the economy than iron filings can; and there is no more reason for taking the one into the system in this crude form than there is for taking the other"

The bad effects of salt are not generally known to those fond of its use at the table. Common salt is a very stable substance that cannot be digested or broken up or utilized by our system. It is excreted unchanged. Every cell in the system coming in contact with salt, contracts. In this way it has a general hardening effect on the tissues. It shrivels the blood corpuscles. It obstructs the general circulation and absorption, and disturbs the natural osmosis, or filtering through the mucous and serious membranes.

CONDIMENTS

"It is needless to say that ginger, spices, nutmeg, cinnamon and all that class of condiments, however much they may vary in quality, are stimulating to a greater or lesser degree, and must be put on the list of "things forbidden" in the hygienic dietary. In doing away with spices and condiments we must also dispense with pickles; there is nothing in a pickle to redeem it from hopeless condemnation. The spices in it are bad, and the vinegar is a seething mass of rottenness, full of animalcules. Mustard is an irritant and a stimulant to the mucous membrane at all times, and for that reason, harmful. The citric acid of the lemon is appropriable by the system, and is one of the most wholesome acids known to us. It will readily take the place of vinegar.
*

The extensive use of spices, salt, vinegar and chemical preservatives in the irrational preparation of our foods, makes them unfit for the formation of healthy blood and tissues. Spices, especially pepper and vinegar, interfere with the formation of red blood corpuscles and, through their constant irritating effect upon the mucous membranes of the intestinal canal, are the chief contributory causes of chronic catarrh and cancer. Salted pickled and spiced foods will insidiously lead to overeating and to the craving for alcoholic beverages". *

*Erz: The Medical Question

COFFEE

Coffee and tea, and to a lesser extent, cocoa, contain poisonous alkaloids which are harmful to the heart, digestive organs, kidneys, brain and nervous system. The caffeine in coffee and the theine in tea are powerful stimulants which cause the heart to beat excessively and irregularly. Caffeine causes a violent excitement of the nervous and vascular systems. Coffee is a drug, a form of dope; and those who habitually use it are, like smokers, drug addicts. Hygienic coffee substitutes, made from figs and cereals, are now in the market. Both tea and coffee retard digestion, as their stimulating effect on the digestive organs benumbs the small stomach nerves. Coffee does not contain any nutritive value. Coffee is an intoxicant; coffee acts directly upon the kidneys, and produces high blood pressure.

The use of tea and coffee causes wakefulness. One cup of coffee will add 700 extra beats to the heart, thus forcing it to work one hour a day overtime. This overwork is paid out of nature's storehouse of vitality. Coffee is a drug, it influences character. Continued use of coffee has a tendency to contract the muscles of the bowels and dry up their natural secretions so necessary to functioning.

The pale, sallow complexion and the inveterate coffee drinker go together. The majority of the world are slaves to one kind of dope or another, and coffee is a form of dope, although coffee is a milder form of cocaine or opium. Coffee drinkers are real addicts through lack of proper knowledge and education of the poisons in it and their terrible nerve-racking and destroying deleterious effects.

TEA

The theine in tea, like caffeine, is very injurious to the nervous system, heart and digestive organs. Herb tea, alfalfa tea and honey tea (made from honey and lemon dissolved in hot water) are hygienic tea substitutes. Tea contains a poison known as theine, which corresponds to a similar poison in coffee, known as caffeine. Both are strong poisons.

Half a gram causes a quick pulse, nervous excitement, slight delusion, and lastly a desire for sleep. Small doses cause sleeplessness, irritability of the bladder and bowels, trembling of the extremities, and other signs of cerebral and nervous distress. Both these poisons work havoc with the system, ruining the nervous and mental life, and creating a dependence on stimulants, which may lead to alcoholic and other excesses. These poisons ruin the taste buds, retard proper digestion, cause constipation, and in many ways tend to ruin the constitution. They cannot be too strongly deprecated.

Even cocoa contains injurious alkaloids, analogous to those contained in tea and coffee, and for that reason is to be avoided. Like all hot drinks, it tends to ruin the taste buds and induces a desire for more food than is needed.

TOBACCO

Tobacco, containing the violent poison nicotine, has a narcotic effect upon the higher cerebral centers and the nervous system in general, seriously injuring the heart, lungs muscles and digestive organs, retarding normal development and leading to premature physical and mental decline.

Smoking interferes with the process of oxidation and the renewal of tissues, and has a most deleterious effect upon the female genital organs, causing pathological conditions in them (when either the woman herself smokes or her husband).

Nicotine is a form of dope; it paralyzes the nerves and deadens the brain. Its persistent use leads to neurasthenia and insanity. Tobacco tends to poison and paralyze the generating organs of both sexes and often kills the seed. It is a law of animal economy that no part of the system can be stimulated or abused, without an expense or tax being placed on the remaining organs. The exhilaration or narcotizing of brain and nerve by the use of alcohol and tobacco are gained at the terrible cost of loss of sexual powers. Tobacco introduces a rank poison into the system. The glands are peculiarly sympathetic with all other parts of the body, and all become poisoned, the testicle gland particularly.

Nicotine destroys the function of the inhibitory nerve that

controls the heart action, also destroying the function of the brain cells. The cellular tissue is saturated with nicotine, appearing in the form of little stationary knots in the tissue, often producing a tobacco heart. Smoking, like drinking, goes hand in hand with meat-eating. The adoption of a vegetarian diet causes one to lose the desire for both tobacco or alcohol, for the irritated and restless condition, induced by meat, which these narcotics were taken to appease, no longer exists.

ALCOHOL

Alcohol, in any quantity and in any form, either as whiskey, wine or beer, poisons the heart, liver, kidneys and nervous system, arousing morbid sex tendencies and causing a gradual degeneration of the brain. The drinking of much alcohol produces marked effects; the taking of a small quantity leads to less noticeable ones. The latter, if accumulated for a sufficient length of time, will, however, make themselves manifest in the form of pathological and degenerative process. Senile dementia (which is an aggravated form of ordinary senility) is such an after-effect of chronic alcoholism.

The use of alcohol cause heart failure, hardening of the arteries, liver and kidney diseases, rheumatism, obesity, high blood pressure and insanity. The pathological effects of alcohol, especially when old age approaches, are very similar to those of meat, except that they are more severe. General physical and mental degeneration, with marked waning of the intellectual faculties, are the final results of the alcohol habit.

Commentary by **LIQUID METAL**

Most people have a few pounds of putrefied feces in their colon. Many people consume organic healthy foods, but most of the nutrients of the foods they eat are wasted. The walls of their intestines are loaded with putrefied waste matter. The way to perfect health is to cleanse your bowels with raw fruit/vegetable diet and fasting.

Speaking of tea, the commercial teas in little bags that you buy in stores or the ones you consume when you go to restaurants or other places, are harmful, no doubt about it. The more you mingle with a natural food, meaning that the further away a product is from its original and natural form, the less healthy it is, or more harmful. I grow my own herbal teas such as sage, mint, lemon balm, chocolate mint etc. I dehydrate them in a dehydrator. If you want my advice, if you like tea (you must only consume herbal ones, any non-herbal one is poison), buy a dehydrator, it is worth it, you can also dehydrate different kinds of fruit or vegetables. Or don't drink teas at all. It's up to you.

Since tea and coffee retard digestion, if you seldom drink them, at least drink them a few hours after the food you consumed has been digested. A lot of foods and drinks that we consume have become so normalized in our way of life that when we read information such as in this book, which recommends to not consume what we deem normal, we might think "What are we going to eat then, grass?" Well, there are many fruit and vegetables that we can eat. You can make fruit cake, or ice cream from fruit. And if you think that flour is needed to make the cake or a pie, you can grind corn, lentils or chickpeas into flour. Sure, it takes effort, but it is worth it. Or if you are strong enough, simply consume fruit, vegetables, seeds and nuts in their original unchanged form.

I consume only herbal tea. I grow it myself. Even if you don't have much land to garden or no land at all, even if you live in an apartment, in the balcony you can plant herbal tea in pots/containers. Just this summer (2024) alone, I harvested enough herbal tea (mint, chocolate mint, sage, lemon balm) to last me a whole year, if not for two years. All these were planted in pots, I harvested twice within the same season. The more you trim/prune them down, the bushier they will grow.

I also dehydrate fig, peach, strawberry, raspberry leaves from the trees/plants I have planted and make tea out of them. You can grow strawberries once, and they grow by themselves every year. Of course, you must propagate them. But with a little effort you can grow your own food or any amount based on each individual's circumstances/needs.

If you are still consuming meat (dead flesh), alcohol, processed foods etc., tea is the least of your worries, assuming that tea is bad. Do not be confused, there is fake/unnatural tea and there is natural herbal tea. But for something to be called natural, means that the product should be in its original state and not processed at all. One example is bread. Bread main ingredient is flour which derives from wheat which comes from the ground. Not only that the modern wheat is poisoned from the spraying of pesticides and the depleted of nutrient soil, but even if wheat was perfectly healthy, by the time it turns into bread, it is not wheat anymore. Bread is processed food, it has salt, sugar, yeast and in most cases cheap harmful oil (which is not fit for human consumption) in it. It is cooked processed product.

The same applies about salt, there is fake/table salt and there is real sea salt.

I showed this chapter to a few friends and they all complained, one said "I love my black tea, I won't let it go" another friend said, "Coffee is my life, there is no way that I will stop drinking coffee". I was like, "Nobody said you should stop doing drugs, I'm simply presenting information, what you do with it, it is up to you". Bread was the last thing that I was addicted to, and I finally let it go, my health improved tenfold.

Because we use the word "*sugar*" to describe the sweetness in fruit, we get tricked into thinking that the sugar from natural fruit is harmful. It is not harmful.

I have consumed a lot of sugar in my life until a few years ago when I began the process of cleansing my body. Your body is designed to protect the internal organs first. So, the system will push out toxins through the skin, exhaling, and rectally first, and anything else that it can't push out from overworking too much, it will direct the toxins at the ligaments for the purpose of saving the internal organs.

For a few years I felt like someone was sticking needles inside my knees, especially when I was going up the stairs. That's because there was too much crystallization of poisons/toxins etc. accumulated in the knees. And the crystallized particles rub against the flesh, bone and anything else within the knee, ankle or any other ligament. When I began my veganism diet, after just a few days I saw a big difference until I stopped having any pain or discomfort anywhere in the body. But this is just my experience.

700 EXTRA BEATS PER DAY WILL NOT MAKE THE MAINSTREAM DOCTORS GO AWAY

Let's do some quick math:

1 hour x **365** days=365
700 x 365=255,500

If you just have one cup of coffee per day, in one year alone, you will add 255,500 unneeded extra beats to your heart. These beats will be taken out of your life force/lifespan reservoir. Unless you are already a superman or a superwoman, having a cup of coffee per day, will shave off years of your life. Pretty much all of us, when we are young and without any health problems, we tend to dismiss, ridicule or deny information that could help us avoid future death/early aging. We think, just because we don't have any pain in the moment, we are fine. But the damage that unhealthy eating and drinking cause is accumulative. The consequences of coffee drinking are detrimental compared to the so-called its benefits.

I have coffee at home, but I don't throw it away. I keep where I see it all the time. This way I test myself and see how strong mentally I am. Not only visually, but I even undo the lid of the jar and smell it sometimes and test my mental power.

Sometimes I hear people saying that *"he or she, lived to 90 or 100 years of age while consuming coffee all life"*. First of all, how do you know someone lived to that age while consuming coffee, did someone told you, did you read it in a book, online or a magazine that promotes coffee drinking? Know that many stories are fabricated for marketing purposes. In many women's magazines about beauty, they advertise all sorts of chemicals and creams for women to put on their skin, losing weight articles, but also they advertise sweets. Isn't that hilarious? Magazines/movies (some have good messages/lessons) have one sole purpose, to keep you weak, sick and to make you age faster, and of course to copy celebrities, so pretty much to keep you distracted and away from your true divine self.

Let's get back to coffee. Even if you knew someone that drank coffee all life, was it a commercial coffee or from an organic nutrient dense soil one? Was it naturally decaffeinated? The person that had coffee all life, was he perhaps a **farmer/gardener*** that maybe he or she was living a **vegetarian*** diet where the only toxic drink he or she consumed was coffee? We are very complicated species. It is false to assume that because someone who has consumed coffee for 70 or 80 years indicates that coffee is healthy. The false assumptions are also based on the belief that living to a 100 years of age is something to be proud of. Before we degraded as a species we lived for hundreds of years. Don't believe the fabricated mainstream history which says that our lifespan is the longest it has ever been. Our species is the most degraded one ever.

Currently I am living a vegetarian/vegan lifestyle. Vegetarian or vegan means natural raw food diet. Any other explanation is false.

A lot of people follow trends without understanding what they're getting into. A lot of store-bought packaged foods say they are vegan, while in reality they are toxic foods, loaded with unhygienic ingredients. One more time, vegetarian/vegan food means raw fruit, vegetables, seeds, herbs and nuts.

If you are a meat eater, it is a big step for you to go on vegetarian diet. If someone told me that living on just air (Breatharianism) is the way to perfect health and immortality, I would be like, "Are you crazy, how can I survive without eating at all?". Fortunately, we are in times where knowledge is available for all who seek it. Step by step is the way to go. Doing the same thing over and over and expecting a different result is not intelligence. If we want change, then we must also change our thinking which it will then lead in changing our actions, in this case lifestyle.

There are 5 stages from complete 100% health to 100% complete decay and vice versa. These stages are:

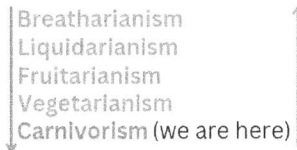

Breatharianism
Liquidarianism
Fruitarianism
Vegetarianism
Carnivorism (we are here)

Check all the words except "carnivorism". They all have the word "Aryan" in it. Aryan means pure. Purity means life. Through propaganda, Nazism many times has been portrayed as the evil ideology that wanted to create a new race called "the Aryan race". Go back further in time, and you will find out that Aryan means pure, AR=Gold, Light etc.

I'm going a little bit off topic here but, a few times I have heard people saying, "If America didn't beat the Germans in WWII, we would all be speaking in German language now". First of all, Germany never lost (*check Operation PAPERCLIP*). Modern America is Germany 2.0. People lost, people like you and me, no matter the nationality. Did 'speaking English' bring us any freedom or peace? There cannot be peace when we remain ignorant of our abilities and powers that we possess.

It's about time to go beyond the surface thinking and focus on what matters the most, which is our physical, mental, emotional and spiritual health. The only way that nobody can control you.

Currently the law of correspondence is imbalanced hence the decay. The Hermetic Law of correspondence works as it should at all times. What we do with our choices comes back to us tenfold. Before mankind began to deteriorate, we were Breatharians. The ether was pure, all we needed was simply oxygen and that's it. But because we were too curious we were like, "let's see what would happen if we drink liquids". And we were like "Wow, it feels good". Eventually, we were like "Oh, look at those colorful things on the plants and trees, lets put them in our mouths and see if they taste good". Again, we were awed at the amazing taste of the fruits and vegetables. As time went by, we saw four legged things roaming around and were like *"Cmon, let's chase them and try to eat them"* and that's when we entered the fifth and last stage of decay, carnivorism.

Carnivorism sealed the deal, the end of our species. I cannot speak for Dr. Bernard, I can speak only for myself, you can do with this information as you please, I did not put this book together to convince you on anything. You life is yours and yours alone, you get rewarded or punished by your own choices. The reaction of your choices is the Universal law that is in place to ensure survival and balance of creation. So, no matter how much we abuse our bodies and nature (including animals), the Universal Laws will make sure that correction of our ignorant and arrogant choices takes place. Correction means "early death", making space for souls that want to master the laws of nature.

> *"Creation will never cease to exist. Only civilizations come and go, but the Creation itself won't go anywhere. We are like fleas that can be shaken off like dust".* – Liquid Metal

You are not responsible only for yourself, but also for you children and their children. Think about it all you want. In case you don't know what this means, read about the 7 hermetic principles and you will understand how our choices affect every single one of the future generations.

"When food that is toxic enters the colon, it is covered by a mucus film for the purpose of holding the toxic substance in suspension, until it is eliminated from the colon. This mucus is sticky and will stick to the colon wall. When a person has a slow-moving colon, this mucus has more time to become stuck on the colon wall, also giving the waste material more time to decay and to begin rotting. This decayed matter will also stick to

the colon wall creating a perfect breeding place for bacteria and parasites to live. Also know that the colon is the organ that absorbs the moisture that goes into the bloodstream. When a person does not drink the proper amount of water to flush the colon, the waste material lays in it and becomes packed and stretches the colon out of shape" – J.Justice, page 395 in his/her book, *"DNA IN THE SANDS OF TIME"*

VEGETARIAN* - Any time you read in this book the word "vegetarian" it means vegan like we use it in our modern day. There shouldn't be a term describing someone that doesn't consume meat but it eats its byproducts (milk, eggs etc.). Either you are vegetarian (fruits, vegetables, herbs, seeds and nuts) or not. People have fallen for certain terms, this way it creates confusion among them.

For a long time I was lying to myself by identifying as a vegetarian while drinking milk (full of puss and antibiotics, let alone that milk is only for the babies of that animal) and consuming eggs (abortion). I was lying to myself, it felt good to think I was vegetarian but my actions (based on ignorance) proved otherwise.

FARMER/GARDENER* – That a farmer or a gardener lives longer than someone who lives in the city or in a fast paced, full of worries and fear life, cannot be debated. Not only that a farmer or a gardener or a person that spend most of his or her time in nature (beach, mountains, forests etc.) is breathing pure electromagnetism, away from city's smog, but someone that spends a lot of time in nature, is not lured into the lust trap.

At home, you are surrounded by technological devices where sexualization is everywhere, even if it's in a soft form, it's still detrimental. Personally I have beaten my sexual urges, so, no more being controlled by lust. But speaking of the garden, in the summer, most of my time is spent planting and tending the garden. I don't think about sex at all. Not that I think when I'm not gardening, but when I'm in nature, my whole being is fully connected with divine Nature/Creation.

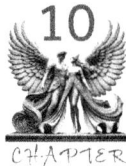

VITAMINS AND ORGANIC MINERALS. CANNED FOODS. WATER; THE PHYSIOLOGICAL FUNCTIONS OF THE ORGANIC MINERALS

VITAMINS AND ORGANIC MINERALS ARE THE MOST ESSENTIAL ELEMENTS IN NUTRITION. While protein supplies nitrogenous material for the support of muscular tissues, and while carbohydrates and fat provides the carbonaceous compounds to produce heat, it is the organic minerals which are required for the activity and well-being of the principal internal organs. These minerals may only be assimilated in an organic form, when in combination with living plant tissue, not in the inorganic form in which they are found in the earth.

In raw vegetables and fruit, these organic minerals are present in combination with absorbed solar energy, or vitamins. These vitamins exist only in combination with organic minerals. Indeed, they are really these very minerals when vitalized by solar electricity; they are manifestations of the complex molecular structures into which these minerals are then organized. As soon as these are broken up by the action of heat, and are resolved into simpler inorganic molecules, the "vitamins" disappear.

WHY COOKED FOODS ARE UNHYGIENIC
Heat above the boiling point, breaks up the loose affinity of the atoms

of the organic molecule, causing the escape of the solar force (the vitamins) contained therein, and converts the minerals into a more stable, inorganic form, in which condition they are unassimilable. In the case of vegetables, these organic minerals are the most important elements they contain, and which the body needs. Cooked spinach, which is recommended so highly, contains no organic minerals whatsoever; and is therefore valueless as an article of food. Its minerals have been rendered inorganic, and have the same injurious effects as a drug containing inorganic iron. The same applies to all other cooked vegetables.

The process of cooking dissolves, precipitates and renders inorganic the minerals contained in vegetables, while destroying their vitamins. Baking produces similar effects. Therefore all cooked foods are injurious; the minerals they contain are unassimilable and poisonous. Besides, cooked foods are minus the vital force present in raw foods (the vitamins), which prevents fermentation. Therefore, when they are taken into the intestines, they rapidly decay, injuring the mucous lining of the digestive tract and forming toxins in the blood.

Cooked food is dead. Raw food, on the other hand, is living. By supplying new cells, which are continually being formed with raw living food, the body may be kept in a state of perpetual youth, Old age is due to an accumulation of impurities in the body, passed on from old cells to new ones. A raw diet will cleanse the organism of these impurities. It will prevent and cure old age.

CANNED FOODS

Canned foods are unhygienic. This is so because of the fact that their minerals have been rendered inorganic and their vitamins have been destroyed by the high temperature to which they were heated. The tin of the can easily passes into solution, particularly when the contents are acid, as in the case of tomatoes and pineapples. Fruits and vegetables of all kinds are now being scientifically preserved by being dehydrated or sun-dried, whereby their minerals are retained in organic form.

WATER

Mineral waters, like drugs, since they contain inorganic, not organic minerals, are injurious. They are unassimilable and settle in the body as calcareous deposits. Water from underground sources (from wells), which contains lime and other inorganic minerals, is unhealthy. Such lime cannot be used to form bones; it causes hardening of the arteries. Of all forms of water, mountain spring water is the best, but not as pure as the water in fruits and vegetables. Water passing through lead pipes dissolves small quantities of poisonous inorganic lead, which has a harmful effect upon the spinal column.

THE PHYSIOLOGICAL FUNCTIONS OF
THE ORGANIC MINERALS

In the past, the organic minerals were considered as nutritive elements of minor importance; in textbooks on dietetics they were termed *"ash"*. However, we are now discovering that they are the most important elements in nutrition. If they are absent, or deficient, no matter how much food a person eats, he will be half starved. This is so because the ductless glands, which govern cell-metabolism and the well-being of all organs, are dependent upon these organic minerals. Without them, they cannot produce their secretions. The thyroid glands for instance, require iodine; the pancreas, silicon. Most people are literally starving to death, though overeating, because of a deficiency of these organic minerals in the diet. Organic minerals are contained in raw vegetables and fruit.

Otto Carque in his "Natural Foods" writes: *"Although the organic salts constitute only a comparatively small amount of the body, about 5%, they hold, nevertheless, the key to nearly all of the material manifestations of life; they are the builders of sound and normal cells and tissues, giving them firmness and form. They are conveyors of vital electricity and magnetism, constantly recharging the human dynamo. They are carriers of life-giving oxygen to all the cells of the body, removing at the same time the products of oxidation. They are essential factors in digestion and assimilation and important ingredients of the digestive juices, regulating the osmotic exchange between lymph and blood and cells. In short, they are indispensable for the proper functioning of all the organs and glands, as well as of the nervous system"*.

The chemical reactions in the cells, which constitute the physical basis of life, take place between substances in solution, and it is by means of the electrical charges carried by these salts in solution that normal chemical reactions in the cells are possible. Through their peculiar electro-chemical attributes, the organic salts maintain, therefore, a very important relation to practically all of the vital processes, for they enter into the composition of every tissue, of all the digestive fluids and of the secretions of the various glands, keeping the proper balance between assimilation and elimination, thus insuring the normal development and functioning of the organism.

The principal organic minerals, which are the constituents of the human body as well as of raw vegetables and fruit, may be divided into two groups, the alkaline and the acid-forming. The former include **potassium, sodium, calcium, magnesium, iron** and **manganese**; the latter, **phosphorus, sulphur, silicon, chlorine, fluorine** and **iodine**. These twelve elements, in addition to oxygen, hydrogen, carbon and nitrogen, constitute the physiological "building stones" of the human body. Every raw vegetable and fruit contains, in different proportions, all of these organic minerals. Some have more of one, some have more of another.

POTASSIUM, and element required by the liver (for glycogen-formation), muscles, red blood corpuscles and brain; is present in high concentrations in all fruits and vegetables. **Tomatoes** contain more potassium than any other member of the vegetable kingdom. Kale, rhubarb and celery are also rich in potassium.

SODIUM, which is required for the neutralization of carbonic acid in the lungs, for the formation of saliva, for the conduction of electro-chemical currents in blood and lymph, and (as a constituent of bile) for the emulsification of fats, is found in greatest quantities in **celery**; spinach, swiss chard, tomatoes, radishes, strawberries, asparagus, carrots, leeks, lettuce, figs and apples are next richest in sodium.

CALCIUM, which is needed for the formation of teeth and bones, for the production of red blood corpuscles, for respiration and for the beating of the heart, is present in greatest concentration in **cabbage**. Dill, lettuce, dandelion, spinach, turnips, lemons and oranges are also rich in calcium.

MAGNESIUM, which is found in the lungs, muscles, brain and bones (giving hardness to the skeleton), is found in largest quantities in **tomatoes**, but also in spinach, lettuce, dill, dandelion and cabbage.

IRON, which, as a constituent of the hemoglobin of the red blood corpuscles, is essential for respiration and oxidation, is contained in largest concentrations in **lettuce**; leeks, spinach, strawberries, radishes, swiss chard, onions, artichoke, cucumbers, tomatoes, plums, celery, carrots, cherries, and grapes are also rich in iron.

MANGANESE is contained in the red blood corpuscles. It is found together with iron, and has similar functions to perform.

PHOSPHORUS is the element chiefly required by the brain and nervous system, being also an essential constituent of the nucleo-proteins of muscular tissue of the bones and of seminal fluid. The food richest in phosphorus is **kale**, next come radishes (large), water cress, sorrel, pumpkins, cucumbers, brussel sprouts and cauliflower.

SULPHUR is a constituent of the hemoglobin of the protein of all tissues and of the sulphuric acid salts which have an antiseptic influence in the alimentary canal. **Kale** contains the most sulphur. Brussel sprouts, dill, watercress, cabbage and cauliflower are also rich in this element.

SILICON is found in muscular tissues, hair, nails and pancreas (as silicic acid). **Lettuce** is richest in silicon. Dandelion, parsnips, cucumbers, onions and spinach are also rich in this element.

CHLORINE is an essential ingredient of the hydrochloric acid of the stomach and the sodium chloride of the blood. **Tomatoes** contain the most chlorine. Celery, dill, lettuce, spinach, kale, radishes, parsnips, carrots and cabbage are also rich in chlorine.

FLUORINE is an important constituent of the enamel of the teeth and the iris of the eye.

IODINE is required for the production of tyrosine/thyroxine by the thyroid gland. It is contained in greatest quantities in **sea-plants, pineapples, garlic, beets, leeks and red onions**.

Commentary by **LIQUID METAL**

No matter how good a cooked food tastes, if it's food that heat reached beyond the boiling point, the vitamins/solar lifeforce is gone. First, avoid drinking tap water, and second, if you have to buy water, make sure it is in glass bottle and make sure that the water is actually from the spring. Don't be deceived by the big wording letters in the front of water package where it says, "Spring Water". Chances are that "Spring Water" is the name of the water company.

Many companies name themselves by putting the words "natural, organic etc." in their name brand to deceive customers into thinking their products is natural and healthy. If a product (food or drink) is packaged in plastic bottles, it is cancerous or unhygienic product, no matter what the ingredients or the wordings in the front of the package says. A greedy company/business that doesn't care about your health would choose the cheapest possible packaging of the product.

Sulphur, chlorine, fluorine (may make you associate it with fluoride) etc. are words that are similar or the same in-house cleaning products. Do not be confused, those are synthetic chemicals in the cleaning products, while the ones listed here are organic minerals produced by your body and nature in its most organic/original form.

If you are someone that consumes cooked food regularly, it is very difficult to stop it, so do it gradually. If you must eat cooked food, eat one meal a day. The other meal or two within the same day make sure it's abundant of fruit and vegetables, because you need the minerals daily. You must be strong. If you decide to consume only raw food tomorrow, don't be swayed by cooked food you may see on Tv, on the road if you pass by a restaurant, or by someone in the house that may be cooking. Don't give in.

If you think you can't let go of something, it's not you, but the parasites in you. And by cooked foods I mean cooked vegetables such as stir-fried or soup. Any other cooked food (pasta, pizza, pies etc.) are completely demineralized and unhygienic.

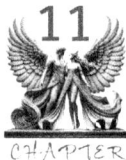

THE HYGIENIC DIET

AS CAN BE SEEN FROM THE 12 ORGANIC MINERALS ANALYSIS, tomatoes are richest in three important organic minerals, potassium, magnesium and chlorine. They also have high concentration of the other minerals, as well as of vitamins A, B and C. Because of their health-giving properties, tomatoes should be used in much greater quantities than they are at present. They should be given to children to be eaten whole, as a fruit, several at a meal.

Foods may be divided in two classes:

One – **Mucous forming**: Those which generate acid-toxins in the blood, which are excreted as mucous or deposited as pus. These foods include (in the order of their mucous-forming capacity): animal foods, fish, eggs, dairy products grains, dried fruit (such as raisins, figs, prunes and dates), nuts and cooked vegetables.

Two – **Non-mucous forming, or hygienic**: Those which supply the blood with the mineral elements required to carry on vital processes, and which render it alkaline and thus better able to neutralize acid-toxins, and to dissolve and eliminate pus. These foods include only raw vegetable and raw fruit.

The cow, and other herbivorous animals live upon the second class of foods, and obtain from them all that is required for the formation of healthy tissue. The human body may do likewise. How does the cow obtain sufficient protein when the grass it eats contains so little of it? This is obtained from atmospheric nitrogen, which is absorbed by the lungs, where, in a similar way as occurs in the leaves of the plants, it is combined with carbon dioxide, phosphorus, sulphur and other elements to form protein. By gradually changing from animal proteins to pot cheese and legumes, and finally to nuts, one may in time entirely dispense with protein foods, and like the cow, obtain all necessary nitrogenous nourishment from the atmosphere.

The old calorie theory was based upon the assumption that we derive heat and energy from the combustion of carbohydrates and fats. This, however, was a false belief. Fasting experiments in which, after a certain day of fast, there was no further loss of weight, without any continued decrease in bodily heat strength and energy, prove that the source of heat and vital power is not the oxidation of carbon compounds, but is the etheric electricity which pours directly and through the nervous system. The human body, therefore, requires no protein or carbohydrate foods.

The only hygienic diet is the one given to man at the beginning, as described in Genesis, composed of raw herbs and fruit. Such a diet will supply the human body with all the elements required for its perfect functioning. However, in most people, the capacity of obtaining protein from the atmosphere, and heat and energy from the ether, is in a very dormant state; consequently a gradual transition from the unnatural to natural diet is required, lets the change involve a too sudden loss of weight. For this reason, fasting is neither beneficial nor advisable – except for the one who has gone through all intermediary steps, and has finally reached the state in which he no longer requires earthly nourishment, but is able to obtain all the elements he requires from atmospheric, etheric and solar sources. (*Dr. Raymond is speaking of "Breatharianism" here, -step 8 in the next page/s-, where all you need to live in perfect health is by simply breathing.* - Liquid Metal.)

One should advance from one to the other of the following diets as fast as the newly awakened nutritive instinct is able to do so, always eating only what is agreeable to the natural sense of taste, and never forcing oneself beyond one's capacity by mere intellectual decision. The dietetic baby must learn to crawl before it may walk. It should not be put upon its feet too suddenly.

Step 1- **THE BLOODLESS DIET**: Consists of eliminating red meat and substituting with white meat, fish and eggs.

Step 2- **THE MEATLESS DIET**: Using fish, eggs and dairy products instead of meat. (L.M - This is what people nowadays call vegetarianism. The word vegetarianism should be used only for raw fruits and vegetables, or anything else that grows on and/or under the ground and not for being a consumerist of animal by products such as eggs, milk etc.)

Step 3- **THE VEGETARIAN DIET**: Eliminating all animal foods, including fish and eggs, using as a substitute fresh pot cheese and legumes. Whole wheat bread should be substituted for white bread, fig-cereal for coffee. Use brown sugar instead of white sugar, and celery salt instead of table salt.

Step 4- **THE RAW FOOD DIET**: This consists only of raw vegetables, fruit, grain and nuts.

For **breakfast**, grapefruit, oranges or melon, or else a fruit salad covered with grated seeds or nuts, should be eaten.

For **lunch**, a raw vegetable salad, composed of cabbage, carrots, cucumbers, lettuce, tomatoes, peppers, green onions, spinach, celery and anise, in different combinations. For those with poor teeth, these vegetables may be ground up together in a juicy, pulpy form by a food chopper. This salad may be seasoned with finely chopped parsley and garlic. It should then be mixed together with ground or grated nuts; and lemon juice and olive oil should be added to it. The above salad, eaten together with unleavened corn bread constitutes a complete meal, and is the surest cure for constipation, as well as of the many diseases which are due to this cause.

Supper should consist of a fruit salad mixed with grated nuts, figs and dates. Or else, the nuts may be eaten together with raisins, figs or dates, and the fruit, including tomatoes, may be eaten whole.

Step 5- **THE RAW VEGETABLE, FRUIT AND SEED-NUT DIET**: This involves substitution of nuts for grains. It is similar to the preceding diet except for the fact that no grains are used. Some may eliminate vegetables, and live on fruits and nuts – finally using no dried fruit, and eating only fresh fruit and nuts.

Step 6- **THE HYGIENIC DIET**: All of the above diets are, to a smaller or greater extent, unhygienic. This is the only truly hygienic one. It contains no mucous forming foods, and consists only of raw vegetables and fruit. This diet will help overcome every disease, for disease are caused by a mucous forming and demineralized diet.

Step 7- THE FRUIT DIET: (Consisting of raw fruit). Vegetables are foods of lower vibration than fruit, and are intended for animals rather than men. As one, in the process of development, acquires an aversion to the eating of animals, so, later , one develops the same feeling concerning the killing and eating of plants.

Step 8- THE COSMIC RAY DIET: This is the diet of the Superman who no longer requires earthly foods, but may obtain this from cosmic radiation alone, the source of all life and nutrition. The sun gives off cosmic rays; and it is these invisible radiations that awaken seeds under the ground to germinate in springtime. So do cosmic rays, generate life electricity in the cells of the human body. While the other diets described above insure greater longevity, only this cosmic ray diet makes possible physical immortality. One meal a day is entirely sufficient. This should be eaten at noon when solar and physiological energy are at their height. Those who have been eating three meals a day, should first eliminate breakfast, then supper.

Commentary by LIQUID METAL

One must gradually change their diet, step by step until one is ready for the final step, the bretharianism or the "Cosmic Ray Diet". Try to follow these four rules when eating:

1- Do not eat fruits and vegetables together
2- Do not drink any liquid with meals
3- Do not eat between meals
4- Give about 5 hours of time between meals

Number 1 is the 1st major hygienic step towards perfect health and immortality. Fruit and vegetables have a different digestion times. Even though the difference is not that big compared when eating fruits/vegetables with cooked foods, it is still bad, for the fact that the food that takes less time to digest will ferment because of the vegetables in this case. And if you consume pizzas (with vegetable topping), or pasta with sauce which contains vegetables, or any other combination where two different foods have different digestion times, your system will be prone to alcoholism. Fermentation is alcohol.

Number 2 - If you drink liquids with meals, the liquid will wash up the digestive enzymes produced in the mouth, the food will end up putting much more stress to your stomach/digestive system. Drink water one hour before eating and one hours after eating, unless you are choking of course.

Number 3 and **4** – There is a process that goes on after you eat, it takes hours. If you eat between meals, you interrupt the process and it resets. Eating snacks is bad, very bad, unless the snack is the meal itself. It goes without saying that by "snack" I mean a carrot, or a vegetable or nuts and not the poisons (crackers, cookies, chocolate bars, pizzas etc.) that the majority of unaware people consume.

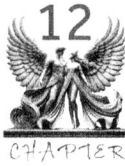

THE CAUSE AND CURE OF DISEASE; THE CURE OF CANCER

TO THE MODERN PHYSIOLOGIST, THE HUMAN BODY is a glandular mechanism. Each organ is under the control of certain ductless glands which activate and energize it by their secretions. Disturbances in any organ are now being traced to a glandular origin, to a deficiency of activating hormones. The medical science of the past has been dealing with effects rather than with the elimination of their internal roots. The medical science of the future will work with the causes, rather than with the effects of diseases. We are now tracing these causes to disturbances of the ductless glands.

The ductless glands are the centers of mineral metabolism. Each of these glands extracts from the blood certain organic minerals, obtained from assimilated foods, transforming these into its secretion, which is then sent back into the blood stream to be carried to certain organs or physiological systems for their invigoration. The normal development, functioning and well-being of these organs entirely depend upon the normal supply of the glandular hormones to which they are sympathetically responsive.

A deficiency or an absence of these hormones will cause them to be weak, devitalized and subject to bacterial infection. Pathologists of the past thought that bacteria were the fundamental cause of organic disease. We now know that this was a false assumption, that bacteria cannot thrive in healthy tissue, any more than can they live in the sunshine, but only where devitalization exists and where rotting matter is present. We have thus far traced physiological disturbances to a glandular origin. When any organ goes wrong, the seat of the trouble is not in that organ but in its ductless gland.

But what determines the condition of the ductless gland?
What causes it to go wrong?

The ductless glands, as centers of mineral metabolism, cannot manufacture their secretions unless they obtain sufficient minerals from the blood. These minerals originally came from the food. If the diet does not contain sufficient amount of these organic minerals, the ductless glands will be starved (no matter how much food is eaten), and the corresponding organs will be devitalized, and consequently diseased.

"The primary cause of disease of death, from a purely physical point, is chiefly mineral starvation due to wrong diet. Indeed, the present diet of the uninformed civilized world is a most perverted one. It consists mainly of flesh, white devitalized flour bread, refined devitalized white sugar and animal fats. That means, it is very poor in the essential organic salts, but very rich in proteins and carbohydrates. People make themselves believe that everything must be cooked, roasted, baked, boiled, salted, spiced and sweetened before it is fit to eat. This unnatural diet overstimulates the system with albumen poisons and carbonic acid gas, which form the basis of all functional derangements and disease"

Since the basic cause of disease is a deficiency of organic minerals in the diet, its cure consists in supplying these to the body through food which are rich in them, such as raw vegetables and fruit. Then the starving ductless glands will obtain the elements they require for the manufacture of their secretions, and the affected organs will be strengthened and vitalized. This will enable them to resist bacterial decomposition, which is only possible while they are in a devitalized condition. The symptoms will then disappear, and the disease will come to an end. Already, we have cured *beriberi* and *rickets* in this rational way. The time will come when every disease will be done away with by such simple means, by removing its fundamental dietetic cause.

(By cleansing the internal enviroment, your electromagnetic field
or aura becomes strong, and no disease can touch you. - L.M)

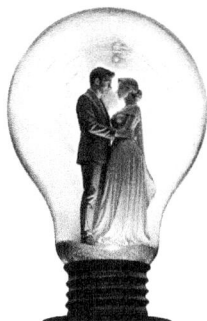

THE FALLACY OF THE GERM THEORY

From this point of view, we can see the folly of trying to overcome disease by inhibiting the activity of the bacteria through antitoxins. This temporary suppression of symptoms does not remove the basic cause of trouble, the presence in the body of rotting waste matter, the decomposition and removal of which the bacteria were effecting. This morbid matter originally came from wrong food. Disease is nothing but a vicarious elimination of waste matter. Pathology is the study of the different ways in which this waste matter is eliminated. The fundamental cause of disease is toxemia, the saturation of the blood with acids coming from mucous-forming foods.

The true physician is not concerned with the superficial removal of symptoms, but with the elimination of their cause, which may only be accomplished by a purification of blood. Through a raw vegetable and fruit diet (for chronic conditions), or a diet of raw vegetable and fruit juices (for acute conditions), he neutralizes the acid-toxins in the blood by rendering it alkaline. By internal irrigation, he gives the intestinal tract a thorough cleansing, to inhibit the formation of more toxins. Chemical laxatives, such as milk of magnesia, should never be used, for these absorb water from the blood, resulting in a higher concentration of toxins within it.

The physician who "fights" against a disease, fights against the body's efforts to cure itself, for disease is not a malignant entity (it is not due to invasion by antagonistic "evil spirits", or their modern equivalent, germs), but is a natural process of physiological self-purification, an elimination of excessive waste matter beyond that of which the excretory organs can normally dispose. The above description applies particularly to acute disease. Chronic diseases partake more of the nature of slow mineral starvation.

Professor Rudolph Virchow, the great German physiologist, said: *"Too much stress is being laid upon the 'germ theory'. Micro organisms are usually found where there is disease; they are also found where there is no disease ascertainable. Hence, microbes may be the result and not the cause of disease. If I could live my life over again, I would devote it to proving that germs seek their natural habitat, diseased tissue, rather than being the cause of the diseased tissue"*

Vaccination, like the administration of antitoxins, is, therefore, an irrational, dangerous and pernicious practice. It is often the direct cause of syphilis, tuberculosis, erysipelas, scrofula, cancer, lymphatic poisoning and epidemics of smallpox itself. It has caused innumerable death of infants and children. Those whom it has not killed, it has poisoned for life. By keeping pure the child's blood, through hygienic food, fresh air and sunshine, lasting immunity to smallpox, as well as to every other disease may be guaranteed. Vaccination, on the other hand, fills the blood with poisonous matter (pus obtained from the sores of a syphilitic animal) which leads to a great number of diseases, including smallpox.

Smallpox is a skin disease, due to unsanitary conditions and to bad food, not to germs. The cowpox which Jenner observed, was a disease in the animal obtained from a syphilitic milkmaid. Epidemics are not fundamentally due to bacteria, but to an **unhealthy condition of large number of people**, as a result of uninformly bad food, living conditions and climate.

You can never catch a disease from someone else. But because majority of people are dying from the inside, by having an unhygienic and rotting internal body/system, some people, when they get sick, it makes them or others think/believe that they got it from someone else. There is no contagious diseases, if there was, none of us would be alive. There is only an internal pollution". – Liquid Metal

Tonsils are lymphatic glands which filter out impurities from the blood. Their enlargement is due to the fact that the system is filled with toxic matter coming from the wrong food (such as bread, cereals, white sugar, dairy products, ice cream, meat, chicken, fish and eggs). The removal of the tonsils deprives the body of an important glandular organ, resulting in the retardation of normal development after puberty, for the tonsils are intimately connected with the sex and thyroid glands. By purifying the blood through a fruit diet, this morbid matter in the tonsils may be re-dissolved and eliminated.

Most operations are both unnecessary and injurious. Pus is not generated by bacteria, but is precipitated from the blood, coming from bad food. By eating no more pus-forming food, and by rendering the blood alkaline through a raw vegetable and fruit diet, the toxic substance which has been previously precipitated may be dissolved again and carried to the organs of elimination. Every abscess and growth in the body may in this way be made to disappear. Appendicitis is nothing but an acute intestinal obstruction which may be cured without operation by internal irrigation and by fasting on fruit juices.

> **❝**
> All medicines are inorganic poisons. While they temporarily remove outer symptoms, they cause worse internal conditions. The apparent curative effect of a drug is due to the fact that after it is taken, the vital force ceases expelling morbid matter (which expulsion appears as the external symptoms) in order to expel the more poisonous inorganic medicine.
> — Cure from within

Thomas Edison said, "The doctor of the future will not dose us with drugs, but will instruct his patients as to the cause and prevention of all maladies". The Greek god of healing, Asclepiades, "Rejecting the use of medicaments, reduced all cure to the order of the diet".

Decaying teeth are caused by an acid blood, due to the use of meat, white flour, and similar foods which are deficient in organic minerals. Dentists are entirely unnecessary, except to relieve people of excess money. Cavities are not due to bacterial action from without, but to an internal dissolving of dental lime by acids in the blood. A natural diet rich in alkaline minerals, will both prevent and cure the decay of teeth without necessitating external treatment.

Cavities should not be filled with metal; the acid blood dissolves this metal, and forms pus underneath. Toothpaste, tooth powder and the toothbrush are unhygienic. No chemical should ever be put in the mouth. The best way to clean the teeth is with a slice of lemon, which is a natural antiseptic. The daily use of raw cabbage will supply the blood with lime to form strong and healthy teeth. Sugar dissolves the calcium of the teeth; therefore it should not be eaten if cavities are to be avoided.

Soap made from chemicals and animal fats should never be used on the skin, for it dissolves the latter's natural oil and abnormally dries the skin. Hot baths, by causing excessive relaxation of the muscles of the pores, injure the skin; and therefore, should seldom, if ever, be taken. A daily cold bath, followed by a brisk massage of the entire body (including the scalp) with the hands, will keep the skin in perfect condition. Sun baths are very beneficial, for they not only vitalize the blood and nervous system, but cause impurities to be given off through the skin. All skin diseases, pimples and boils are do to wrong food, and may be cured by raw vegetable and fruit diet.

The falling out of hair is due to a lack of mineral in the diet, to the wearing of a hat, to too frequent washing and to cutting. The hair, like every other part of the body, has a vital function to perform; it acts as an antenna, absorbing electrical energy from the ether for the invigoration of the nervous system. The cutting and shaving of the hair deprives the body of this power, as illustrated by the story of Samson. Eye trouble is due to a diet deficient in organic mineral, sexual excess and overstrain. The eyes may be cured without the use of glasses by a hygienic diet, by continence and by contact with the soothing green color of nature.

THE CURE OF CANCER

Cancer is a cellular derangement caused by a demineralized diet. Certain cells, starving for organic minerals, feed upon other cells, in order to obtain them. A similar process occurs when a pregnant woman's diet does not contain enough calcium for both herself and the embryo; the latter will obtain this from her own bones and teeth, which will then be dissolved. So, the entire organism of the cancer patient is fed upon by starving cells. The parasitic cells increase in size, while the other diminish. The chemical equilibrium of the blood is thus disturbed; and a certain inhabitation which tends to limit cell growth is removed. The parasitic cells grow to tremendous proportions, reproducing prolifically, and filling the blood with their progeny.

Experience has proven that X-ray treatment and operation cannot cure cancer. The cure of cancer is not a local but a general one; it is a matter of blood chemistry. The fundamental cause of the disorder must be removed. This means feeding the starving cells with the minerals they require. This may be accomplished by a diet of raw vegetables and fruit especially rich in the organic minerals needed by the afflicted organs. The blood then regains its chemical equilibrium, and the parasitic cells are not permitted to grow beyond their normal size, not have they necessity to feed on the others.

Commentary by LIQUID METAL

In modern times, people spend too much time indoors, whether it is at a workplace, schools (indoctrination facilities), malls, or being distracted at home by technological devices. People don't spend enough time outdoors where they can be healed to a certain degree by the Sun alone. Sun is one of the main cures of everything. Just as is fasting or raw food diet. The path to perfect health is a long journey. Step by step, beginning by getting rid of the death/foods and drinks that you consume, practicing chastity, fasting, sun gazing/sunbathing etc. you will glow externally and internally.

If you have a cough, runny nose etc., don't rush in to take pills or any other form of medicine by the mainstream so-called health care system. Let it run its course. If you take medicine, you are simply suppressing the symptoms. When you discharge phlegm from your throat or the nose, don't panic, that's your body that is getting rid of the toxins or any other pathogen. If you suppress that process, then you will continue to have in you those toxins that otherwise would have been eliminated by themselves if you didn't suppress them with temporary medicine. Drink homemade fruit or vegetables juices, or fast (but you must drink while fasting), especially when you have any discomfort, pain, flu etc. Disease cannot touch you if your inner (internal organs, muscles, nervous system etc.) habitat is clean and pure.

THE APENDIX IS USEFUL - CREATION DOESN'T MAKE MISTAKES
The appendix was bothering me until a few years ago when I began cleansing myself, I stopped eating rotten flesh/meat 7 or 8 years ago. Only recently (in the last couple of years) I stopped consuming dairy products. From then I was consuming only raw vegetables, fruit, herbs, seeds, nuts and cooked food, mainly vegetable cooked food, and occasionally spaghetti/pasta, and pizza and bread. I was drinking and still I am only drinking water (not tap water), and occasionally distilled water and home-made fruit juices.

I'm not big on vegetable juices, it seems that my body is inclined more toward fruit. In the last month or so, I stopped consuming cooked food. From the moment I used to consume dead flesh to the moment I consumed my last cooked meal I had progressed a lot, but it's when I began a pure raw fruit and vegetable diet that I saw what real health meant. Now, you may be someone that disagrees, you may be someone that are still attached (actually controlled by the parasites in dead foods) to meat, cooked foods, processed/toxic foods and drinks. If that's the case, you may be disagreeing with a very advanced step.

Do you remember the eight steps from Dr. Bernard, where the eighth step was the COSMIC RAY DIET? Yes, analyze the eight steps. Find where you're at and progress incrementally onto the next step.

The appendix, for too long, was considered a vestigial organ, meaning an organ that lost its original function through evolution. And that was a false assumption as there are many other false assumptions from the mainstream medical mafia. The appendix plays an important role in the immune system by storing and releasing good bacteria that the body uses to flush disease-causing organisms from the intestine. Some people think that taking out the appendix is not a big deal. The human body is neither created with extra organs, nor it is created to waste seminal secretions/semen (including blood and eggs through menstruation).

The cure for cancer is already available in you. Sure, there are other ways to cure it such as through specific vibrational frequencies and certain special pills, but you will get it again (or any other disease) if you continue eating rotten and toxic foods and drinking toxic drinks. There is no easy way to perfect health without effort. Disease starts from within and from within it can be cured.

PART IV

PARTHENOGENESIS
(VIRGIN BIRTH)

&

THE SUPERMAN

How a superman may be Parthenogenically conceived by an electro-Magnetism Fertilization of the Human Ovum.

"Why not try creating a race of Supermen, endowed with physical and intellectual attributes very superior to others? This conception may appear revolutionary at the present time, but there is no reason why such an attempt should not be made" – Dr. Serge Voronoff: *The Conquest of Life*

"Then we shall see only heroes born; and the least of our children will have the strength of Zoroaster, Apollonius or Melchizedek; and most of them will be accomplished as the children Adam would have had by Eve, had he not sinned with her. 'Then, Sir', I continued, 'your Cabala empowers man and woman to create a children otherwise than by the usual method?'
'Assuredly' he replied.
'Ah, Sir' I entreated, 'teach this method to me. I beg of you."

- Monfaucon: Comte de Gabalis

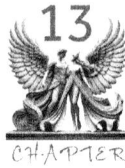

JESUS, AN EUGENIC SUPERMAN

THE ESSENES WERE AN ORDER OF VEGETARIANS, pacifists and mystics, composed of the more intelligent and spiritual members of the Hebrew race, who were later known as the early Christians. That they were more well versed in the science of eugenics than we are today, is illustrated by their scientific regulation of marriage and procreation, and by the fact that many supermen, including Jesus and John the Baptist were produced by them. Having descended from the School of the Prophets, they flourished from 600 B.C. until the beginning of the fourth century, when their opponents and persecutors established the Roman Church and destroyed the communities where they were practicing the pristine, unadulterated teachings of Jesus.

According to the Apocryphal New Testament, two thousands years ago, certain Essene eugenists decided to create a Superman. Accordingly, certain especially qualified individuals were selected as his grandparents, a rabbi named Joachim, and a virgin named Anna. They had both lived chastely since the time of their marriage (more than twenty years before); and, though of very mature age, they still retained their youthful vitality.

For a superman to be produced, it is necessary that his mother be conceived, prenatally cultivated, born and educated in accordance with scientific principles, and under eugenic supervision. Therefore, though Joachim and Anna could not become parents of a superman, they could give birth to a potential mother of one. The eugenists discussed the matter with them; and it was agreed that the resulting child, after its weaning, was to be given over to the care of Essene educators, to be raised under ideal conditions, so that when it reached maturity, it might become a fit parent of a superman.

Under the guidance of Essene eugenists, Joachim and Anna underwent a preparatory training previous to conception, in order to purify their blood and vitalize their bodies so that they might be able to conceive a child in an immaculate manner. This preparation included a forty day fast by Joachim. Thus, in a passionless and spiritual way, in a spirit of service to posterity, Mary was conceived by parents who had lived chastely throughout their lives. The infant Mary was given especial care; her room was kept spotlessly clean, and only virgins and priests were permitted to come near her. Her mother devotedly nursed her for the full period of three years, after which she was given over to the eugenists who had prepared for her coming. She was raised by them, upon a vegetarian diet and in the company of virgins, until she reached maturity.

A certain male among the Essenes, who had been similarly prepared, was selected as the father of the unborn superman; and both Mary and he were instructed by the eugenists how they might conceive a child in a manner other than that usually employed (which, among the Essenes, was called the Immaculate or Pure Conception). So, in a spirit of devotion, devoid of personal emotions, the child Jesus was immaculately conceived. According to an ancient Essene manuscript rescued from the Alexandrian Library (which the founders of the church burned so that all records of the Essenes, and of Jesus' relation to them might be destroyed), and to a section in an eighth century Slavonic edition of Josephus' "History of the Jews" (subsequently omitted), the father of Jesus was an Essene. His so-called disciples, who were not Essenes, show their ignorance of his percentage by tracing his genealogy through Joseph, who was not his father.

It became known that a new superman was in the making. This caused the Roman despots great uneasiness; for, should another Moses appear, the time was ripe for a revolution. Therefore, an order was issued that all newborn male children should be killed. Since the life of the now embryonic Jesus would be in danger if Mary stayed with the Essenes, she had to leave them. That her chastity as well as her safety might be most secure, she was married to an elderly widower, of honourable reputation, named Joseph, who was chosen by the Essenes as her protector. During gestation, Mary lived at the home of Zacharias, high priest of the Temple of Jerusalem, who was one of the eugenists who had supervised her coming into being and her education, while Joseph was in a distant city, building a house. Previous to the time of the child's expected arrival, he returned, and together with his sons, departed with Mary to Egypt. On the way, while Mary was in a cave in the desert, her child was painlessly born.

Commentary by LIQUID METAL

In ancient Lemuria, Atlantis and any other civilization when they were thriving by being fully connected to nature, the women were giving birth through parthenogenesis. They were chaste. They did not menstruate. Back then it was normal that children born were super healthy and intelligent children.

Eventually humanity began to decay. We can see it in our current society. Most children are born incomplete, beginning with their prematurely cut cord. Many mothers, while pregnant, smoke, drink alcohol and/or soft drinks, watch low frequency [horror/blood] content in movies/TV shows, consume processed food, have sex with the father of their unborn child while pregnant etc. All these poisons the blood by interfering with the proper growth of the child. Let alone that most people don't know that a child should be conceived at a specific time of a year based on their zodiacal sign.

To many people, the parthenogenesis subject may be new. Learning more things daily is not necessarily a good thing. The more things you add in your mind, the more you have to think about. Learn to become an observant in life rather than rationalizing.

There is a farmer/gardener I know. All he does in life is about planting, gardening, flowers etc. And he is happy. He knows nothing about politics, conspiracy theories, manifestations/affirmations, spirituality etc. All he does is being engaged in nature. He is connected with it.

Benevolent and malevolent eugenics

Recently on social media, I have seen/read a few times about this subject (parthenogenesis). In two cases, the people that were talking about this in a negative way were women. These women definitely men haters. They were saying "good riddance of men which they don't exist, only women do". Of course, these two have fallen victims of the negative intention about eugenics and/or the evil agenda that is about getting rid of masculinity.

The positive side is to create a species where everyone loves and care about one another. The negative side is to get rid of masculinity, because without men or strong men, societies are easier to control. There are benevolent and malevolent higher forces out there that have always battled against each other for us. The benevolent ones want us to be free and raise children where both parents teach children love, care, peace and freedom. The malevolent beings want to get rid of masculinity and suppress feminine. Don't fall for that agenda. The same applies for the opposite where there are woman haters out there.

In the world there always was, now even more, men and women that are helping others rise and escape from the mental chains. Eugenics is good only if the intention is to bring peace, strength, love and freedom for all. Government means tyranny, but it can also be called leadership (instead of government) if the intention was to help as opposed to suppress us. It is true that when we are conceived, we begin as females first. But so what? Why should it matter? Evil eugenic is when a certain group of beings (tyrannical beings hiding behind the puppets/government officials) eliminate millions of people, especially those that cannot be controlled a.k.a the rebels. Are you a rebel? Are you against tyranny and pro peace and freedom?

A child needs to bond with both parents (masculine and feminine). In my opinion, if you can't conceive a child, do not use the sperm of someone else. In someone else's sperm there is the DNA of that person. That unknown man could have been an alcoholic, a drug addict, a killer etc. It will then transfer to the baby which will then contribute to the reincarnation of the child in 3D reality. If you can't have a child, maybe there is a reason for it.

Someone I know, couldn't bear a child. For years, she had so much free time, she used it to create social media accounts and help humanity awaken. If she had children, perhaps she wouldn't have time to plant seeds of freedom. Listen to your inner voice, it speaks to you at all times, all you got to do is to listen to it. You don't have to do what majority does.

ARE YOUR EARNINGS MORE THAN YOUR HUSBAND OR YOUR WIFE?

Unfortunately, many times in our society, men or women that earn more than their partner, become condescending. Value is not just in money, but also in feelings, thoughts and feminine or masculine presence. Since I have been together with the mother of my children for over 20 years, she always earned more than me. She has two degrees which earns her good money to live comfortable without major concerns. She never used her profession/income against me. As a matter of fact she never needed the money I earned throughout the jobs I have worked at. But she never told me to leave. Why? Because she is a self-ware woman and she fully understands the importance of a father and a man in the house. Just a masculine presence in the house, is safety for her and our children.

A lot of relationships end unnecessarily, because of egoism between couples or other (personal gain – money/sex etc. reason) reasons, but it's the children that pay the ultimate price. Don't fall for "All women are the same or all men are the same". Clearly, not all women or men are the same. If you think that, it means that you have only met people that live in that category. When you meet someone that understands you, that respects and allows you to be free without conditions, then you will clearly see that not all men/women are the same.

If you haven't already done so, never have a child with another woman (or another man if you are a woman reading this). Even if the new woman is the right one and the mother of your child was the so-called bad one. I am advising you to not do this because of the astral pollution that every person has in them.

When you have sex with another person that is not completely clean from previous relationships, she will infect you with the low frequency and DNA of any of her ex boyfriends or husbands. If you made a mistake that you got together with the wrong person, accept it and live with it, meaning that if you divorce, then be alone, be chaste.

Unless you completely clean yourself and get together with someone else who also is 100% clean physically, mentally, emotionally and spiritually, then you can have sex (assuming you don't want to have intelligent children through parthenogenesis) and have average children. Then the child would be a superman or a superwoman (if continence and raw and natural food methods were followed previous to, during pregnancy and after child birth for at least three years).

A superman child is born with ZERO karma to pay. Do you understand why most people are born with amnesia and live a misery life? Because their parents lived a filthy life, meaning consuming meat, sex, alcohol, dairy and other junk food and drinks. What this did to them, was that it caused them to be attached to earthly 3D reality and when they passed away, they were so confused and scared that they chose to come back (reincarnate) in 3d Earth reality again because that what was familiar to them.

But you have knowledge now, practice it so that you don't meet the fate of your parents. When you live a raw food and chaste life, you will be completely clean and when (if) you pass away you will remember all memories of this lifetime, and since now you have this knowledge, you will then decide to be born to parents that also have and practice this knowledge. When you are born to parents that practice chastity and raw food diet, your children also, in the next life will inherit the same knowledge. Long story short, there is a saying,

"If you teach your children the right knowledge, it's as if you've already taught the same knowledge to your grandchildren, even if you never meet your grandchildren".

Have you ever thrown a little snowball down the mountain where the ball gains momentum and it becomes bigger? The same applies if you teach the right knowledge to your children. Their children and all generations after should inherit the same knowledge and more.

THE ANCIENT HEBREW AND HINDU DOCTRINE OF THE IMMACULATE CONCEPTION

THERE HAS BEEN NO GREATER INFLUENCE TO RETARD the evolution of the race than that which has distorted and veiled the profound truths which the Essene doctrine of the Immaculate Conception was originally intended to convey to humanity. That the Immaculate Conception has been made to appear miraculous and supernatural, a solitary event incapable of repetition, and something which every rational and scientific mind must reject as absurd, has prevented the birth of many more individuals of the type of Jesus, and even greater ones, during the last two thousand years.

Jesus was an eugenically-created human. While he was yet unborn, his grandmother and mother, under the directions of Essenes eugenists, devoted their lives to prepare for his coming. If children today will be afforded equally rational eugenic, prenatal, and postnatal conditions as was Jesus, many more such as he will come into being. Mary brought forth her superman child not to show the world an impossibility, as it has been made to appear by the church, but an example for every healthy and normal girl to imitate.

The doctrine of the Immaculate Conception is of ancient Hebrew Origin; it was an essential part of the esoteric teachings of Moses (the Cabala) given too the more spiritual Levites, and handed down by them to the School of Prophets and to the Essenes (who later became the early Christians). That the original sin (symbolized by the eating of the apple) referred to sexual intercourse as distinct from procreation, and that a higher method of generation existed during that early age, is proven by the fact that the words "Adam" and "Eve" signified races rather than individuals (for, since Cain went to the land of Nod, and there found a wife and built a city, many more people must have been living in Adam's day' and these must have reproduced in some way).

Since God commanded man to "be fruitful and multiply", he did not forbid reproduction, which was then accomplished in an immaculate (or electro-magnetic) manner. But what was forbidden was sexual intercourse, the lower animal use of the reproductive function. The eating of the forbidden fruit, and the Fall of Man, can mean nothing else than a descent to an inferior and coaster method of procreation, the generation of children by sexual intercourse rather than by a chaste and immaculate relationship.

The Hindus and Egyptians believed in the Immaculate Conception may centuries before the advent of Jesus. So did the Persians (whose Zoroaster was immaculately conceived) and the Greeks (whose Plato was supposed to have been the child of a virgin). The Hindus believed that Chrishna and Buddha were born from virgin mothers; however, like Zoroaster and Plato, they both had fathers. The following is the Hindu version of the facts related above:

"As in the Golden Age there are no carnal relations between man and woman, so is there none in the Silver Age, although man and woman, as husband and wife, live together in houses, have housekeeping and enjoy material comforts. Yet, strange as it will strike most of you at this distance in time, the Golden Age and Silver Age women bear and give birth to children. The child is born in the womb of its mother at the wish and command of the husband. She has no pain of child-birth to suffer from.

During the Golden Age and the greater portion of the Silver Age, all men and women are, what the Christians call 'virgin-born'. The fuss that is made about this immaculate conception succeeds only to excite a smile of pity in the Shastra-enlightened Hindu – a smile of pity for the ignorance of the facts of the past history of the human race of which they seek to know so little and care less to know more. This fact about the Golden and Silver Ages, this generally prevailing immaculate child conception, ought to open their eyes".

Recent scientific discoveries demonstrate the possibility of an immaculate conception. An unfertilized egg has been made to develop into an embryo by a substitution of electro-magnetic radiations for the spermatozoon. When a man and a woman, whose bodies, as a result hygienic and continent living, are sufficiently charged with vital electricity of opposite polarity to permit a powerful current to flow between them, the human ovum may be parthenogenically stimulated to embryonic development.

This would mean that the human genital organs were never intended by nature for the use of which they are ordinarily being put; and that sexual intercourse is a perversion of a natural function, being nothing else than double masturbation. We cannot expect the superman to be ushered into the world by this means.

THE IMMACULATE CONCEPTION

Since the conception of Mary and John the Baptist, like that of Jesus, were angelically heralded, and since both Mary and John were "filled with the Holy Ghost from their mother's womb", we may believe that they also were immaculately conceived. The Christian sect of the Collyridians believed that Mary was immaculately born from a virgin. Since less care was taken to conceal the true nature of Mary's conception than that of her son, a description of this, as given in the Apocryphal New Testament, will shed some light on the manner in which Jesus was conceived. We find the following concerning the immaculate conception of Mary by Anna and Joachim:

"An angel of the Lord stood by her and said, Anna, the Lord hath heard thy prayer; thou shalt conceive and bring forth, and thy progeny shall be spoken of in all the world. Behold Joachim thy husband is coming with his shepherds. For an angel of the Lord hath also come down to him, and said, 'The Lord God hath heard thy prayer, make haste and go hence, for behold Anna thy wife shall conceive'. And Joachim went down with the shepherds, And she ran, and hanging about his heck, said, 'Now I know the Lord hath greatly blessed me. For behold, I who was a widow am no longer a widow, and I who was barren shall conceive.

The rejoicing at each other's vision, and being fully satisfied in the promise of a child, they gave thanks to the Lord who exalts the humble. After having praised the Lord, they returned home, and lived in a cheerful and assured expectation of the promise of God. So Anna conceived, and brought forth a daughter, and according to the angel's command, the parents did call her name Mary"

In the article "The Immaculate Conception" in the Catholic Encyclopedia, we find the following: "St. John Damascene esteems the supernal influence of God at the conception of Mary to be so comprehensive that he extends it to her parents. He says of them that during the generation they were filled and purified by the Holy Spirit, and freed from sexual concupiscence. Some writers even taught that Mary was born of a virgin and that she was conceived in a miraculous manner when Joachim and Anna met at the golden gate of the temple"

Concerning the conception of Jesus, we read: An angel said to Mary, "While you are a virgin, you shall conceive without sin and bring forth a son" To this discourse of the angel, the virgin replied not, as though she were unbelieving, but willing to know the manner of it. She said, "How can that be? For seeing, according to my vow, I have never known any man, how can I bear a child without the addition of a man's seed?"

To this the angel replied and said, "Think not, Mary, that you shall conceive in the ordinary way. For, without lying with a man, while a virgin, you shall conceive; while a virgin, you shall bring forth; and while a virgin give suck. For the Holy Ghost shall come upon you, and the power of the Most High shall over-shadow you, without any of the heats of lust. So that which shall be born of you shall be only holy, because it only is conceived without sin".

(Reminder, that being born in sin, means to have been born through the ordinary procreation method, which is through 'sexual intercourse'. All of us were born in sin. When you grow all life learning that the only way to procreate is through sexual intercourse between a man and a woman, you would think that any other way of procreation would be nonsense or unbelievable. Depending on your age, whether you know or remember, long time ago, it would take days, or weeks for a mail you had to send to your family across the sea. But now, instantly you can write to anyone, and anywhere in the world through messaging systems, emails etc. So, always be ready to consider what you think is impossible. – L.M)

Alexander the great was immaculately conceived. Nectanebus, and Egyptian prophet and astrologer, his father (who was not Philip of Macedon), said to his mother, Olympias, "I will bring unto thee the gods who came forth from beneath the earth, and they shall come in to thee and they shall hold converse with thee, and then thou wilt get from them that which shall make thee glad. And behold, a son shall be born to thee. If thou desireth that this god should come unto thee in his very person, give me a place near unto thee, wherein I may pray". And Olympias said to him, *"Take then this chamber, which is behind this place, and if I do in very truth become with child, I will honor thee to be the father of the child".*

✴ Commentary by **LIQUID METAL**

There is no 'Jesus' or any external savior to save you, I mean an external physical Jesus. You have the capacity to make the right choices to be and do what he did. Would you want your children all their lives for you to guide them or save them, or would you want them to find their own way? If they waited for you all their lives, they would remain as children, undeveloped without self-aware personal experiences, they would not think for themselves but would rely on external beings or authorities to tell them what to do and how to think.

You too, can raise your frequency to Christ Consciousness level just like Jesus did. There is information out there that Jesus or Yashua never existed. But so what? Every second of the day, you have the opportunity to become greater than you were the day before.

No amount of money or riches can make up for abusing our bodies with filthy food and drinks. The body that we carry with us all day long, is the greatest gift ever given to us. Just think about it, you have a flesh and bones, nervous system, muscles, brain etc. Isn't it amazing to be able to be in one such marvelous technological natural device? Right now, most people are like used and broken down computers, full of viruses (diseases).

As a woman, If you are not cleansed, you cannot bring a super child to this world. But you can bring a potential future mother or father for the next generation of children. We must not be selfish and think only what we can gain in the moment, we must think about the next generation and any other after that. If you continue to abuse your body, you will keep reincarnating without memories of the previous life.

Be careful that you don't get deceived by some articles only about "Parthenogenesis". For everything, there is positive and negative sides to it. There is white magic which creates a superman through chastity and raw food diet where the body is completely clean, and there is black magic, by procreating through the releasing of the seminal fluid through sexual intercourse. Some information out there entices women to hate men and vice versa. They use the information is such subtle and smart deceiving ways that you may fall for it.

Make sure you breastfeed your child for at least 3 years. During pregnancy you must not have sex or anything sexual with the father of the child, and definitely not with anyone else either. Almost all parents say, "My child is fine, nothing wrong with him or her". What is considered a sick child, when he or she limps, or needs a surgery? Many diseases are not visual ones. All of us were born incomplete. Not only that the umbilical cord was prematurely got cut off, but we were also fed junk food and drinks for many years. The sooner we begin to stop lying to ourselves, the sooner we begin to stop lying to our children.

When man ate the forbidden fruit, meaning when mankind began reproducing through sexual intercourse and not through an immaculate relationship, meant that humans initiated the reincarnation cycle. Before that, there was no need to keep incarnating over and over. Whether humans began reincarnation because they were ignorant, not knowing what they were getting into, or whether they were tricked by higher beings with an evil intentions, doesn't matter now. What matter is to begin rising up in spiritual consciousness by cleansing ourselves so that we stop the incarnation cycle.

ADAM AND EVE

Adam & Eve were races of giants beings. They did not consume solid food. They were breatharians, nourished just by the cosmic rays or the ether. They were very tall, up to 100 meters tall. It may seem ridiculous to you but how do you seem to an ant? There were giant trees up to one or even two thousand of meters tall. The giants of those times breathed fresh air.

The higher up you are the more clean and undisturbed ether one would breathe. Not only that people are not giants anymore and live in the cities or crowded areas, but they don't breathe consciously with the diaphragm anymore. When you don't breathe with your diaphragm, your breaths are shorter which means that within a day you would use many more breaths out of your life reservoir of breaths which will then result in a shorter life, no matter how healthy you eat.

We are a very big threat to the beings (you can call them aLIEns if you wish or extraterrestrials, beings form the extra lands beyond Antarctica) that have suppressed mankind's potential for a very long time, since the fall of man; the fall, being that we began:

1- *Procreating through the ordinary method of sexual intercourse.*

2- *Through a solid food diet, until we began consuming dead flesh (carnivorism), which is the lowest level a living and a sentient being (that* *has a thinking brain) can go/fall in consciousness.*

Could the Adam and Eve (giants) races also swim underwater? Have you ever heard of "Mermaids", the aquatic creatures? Could the people that depicted the mermaids with the head of a body of a human and the tail of a fish, depicted them because they saw them swimming as fish? Just as the dormant Kundalini is depicted as a serpent, so other ideas or beings were depicted as different creatures/animals. Could the Mermaids have been the remnants of the giant races or one of the great races?

The beings that suppressed our potential have been working nonstop to suppress our powers through toxic food and drinks, wi-fi, short wave radio signals etc. They shrunk us, we are the descendants of the Giants. The descend didn't happen from 100meter tall to 1.8m. It happened gradually through the course of hundreds and thousands of years.

The more oxygen we breath the bigger we become. But you may ask, "how about people that live in the mountains, why are they not giants? They are too, fallen; what do they eat?" Do they have physical sex? We won't become giants in just one generation. Even though there are people that live in remote areas with better air such as in the mountains or in the woods/forests, they too live in the same Earth (with a hijacked or damaged electromagnetism) that you and me live in.

As of now, this is still a slave realm. Earth was supposed to be a school and not a prison. The population itself is the prisoner and the warden at the same time. Use money to improve your life through reading books, gardening, crafting but don't be its slave by buying materialistic nonsense that enslaves you. Use technology (phone, tablets, internet) to spread truth and help one another, but don't become slave to it where you waste your precious time watching porn, other meaningless pics/videos/information, arguing online with people etc.

PARTHENOGENESIS

ACCORDING TO THE OVISTS, THE FEMALE PARENT is held to afford all of the materials necessary for the formation of the offspring, the male doing no more than awakening the formative powers possessed by, and lying dormant in the female product. This was the theory of Pythagoras, adopted in modified form by Aristotle. Blondel, in his "The Power of the Mother's Imagination over the Fetus" explains as follows the Ovist theory, namely that the egg is a potential embryo:

"All parts of the foetus/fetus, both small and great, internal and external, are in the ovum. And though some appear later than others, yet they have been co-existing, and have had their beginning at the same time – as an acorn, which, even before it be set in the ground, does contain an epitome of the oak, with all its roots, branches and leaves". – Blondel, *The Power of the Mother's Imagination over the Foetus*

In 1762, Bonnet performed parthenogenic experiment which disproved the old theory of the Spermatists (propounded by Galen), that in the male semen there were seeds which entered into the eggs and there developed into embryos; and which supported the ovist theory (as modern parthenogenic experiments now do), that in the ovum, and in the ovum alone, are contained the germinal potentialities of the future organism. As Professor Lester Ward said, "Life begins as female. Life is feminine. In woman is the 'creative center'. That everything proceeds from the egg, the 'vital focus', is the verdict of biology.

The present theory of conception as due to spermatozoa and ova was held by the medical profession only since the middle of the last century. Previous to this time, a theory was held known as the Aura Seminalis theory, according to which the semen of the male does not fertilize the egg by material contact but by an "aura" or radiation it gives off. This theory was subsequently disproven by experiments performed by Spallanzani, repeated by Prevost and Dumas in 1848. According to recent scientific investigations, spermatozoa add no new germinal material to the eggs they fertilize, but act as catalytical agents, chemically stimulating them to cell-division and embryonic growth.

These parthenogenic experiments directly disprove the Weismannian theory of germ-cell inheritance, and demonstrate that organisms which ordinarily reproduce sexually have a latent parthenogenic capacity which improved environmental conditions and appropriate stimuli may evoke.

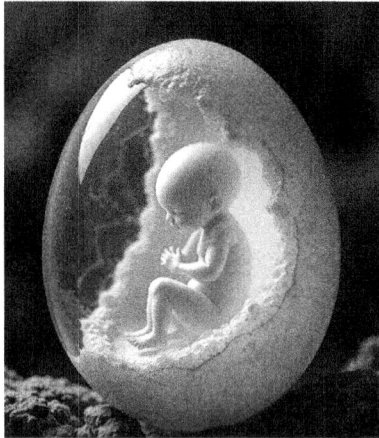

Primordial forms of life all produce parthenogenically; it is only when outer conditions are unfavourable, and when they are devitalized, that they resort to a sexual mode of reproduction. However, as soon as external conditions are improved, and their strength increases, they return to their original parthenogenic method of generation. Since chemical activity is essentially an electrical process, due to charged ions in solution, we may say that fertilization is an electro-magnetic stimulation of the ovum to embryonic development.

This has been proven by biological experiments. "Lillie and Hinrichs of the University of Chicago have virtually created life with rays. The eggs of the sea-urchin when laid by the female must be fertilized by the sperm of the male in order to produce young. These scientists were able to fertilize the eggs with ray alone. As Dr. Hinrichs stated, 'This eliminated the male entirely, for this egg became a swimming fish without the male sperm'. The only father these fish had was radiation".

One of the most remarkable phenomena in the field of parthenogenesis is that of dermoid cysts, the parthenogenesis development of an embryo within the human body.

"It has been demonstrated that these cystic growth contain, unquestionably, the vestigial embryonic remains of human growth, analogous to that of female gestation - hair, teeth, skin, flesh, bones, tissues, glands, portions of the scalp, face, eye, rib, vertebral column, umbilical cord, even the embryonic sac – they are frequently found in virgins or very young females" – Buzzacott, *Mystery of the Sexes*

In Volume VIII of the Reference Handbook of the Medical Sciences, it is stated: "The most characteristic feature of ovarian dermoids and solid teratoma is the fact that they contain tissues derived from all three of the germ layers. Their structure giving the impression of a rudimentary embryo. According to Wilm and others, a parthenogenic development of an unfertilized ovum may be assumed".

That many of these so-called cystic growths may be actually embryos which have been immaculately, or electro-magnetically conceived, to the ignorance of both patient and physician, is illustrated by the following case quoted by Dr. Kisch, in his book, "The Sexual Life of Woman":

"A girl who, in consequence either of actual intercourse or it may be merely of too intimate an embrace of a man, fears she has become pregnant and actually suffers from amenorrhea (cessation of menstruation) though pregnancy does not really exist. I saw a case in which amenorrhea was thus produced in a girl of seventeen years of age, whose ideas on the process of sexual intercourse were still far from clear. She had permitted a young man to kiss her repeatedly and fervently, and to clasp her in close embrace. She was then afraid that she had become pregnant; the catamenial flow, which had been regular since she was fifteen years of age, ceased to appear".

This quotation has ben made not because this case is an authentic instance of immaculate conception, but to demonstrate the fact that there exists in the female an instinctive feeling, which is barely suspected by the male, than an immaculate conception is possible.

🔔 *Commentary by* LIQUID METAL

What if, many times, sexual intercourses resulted in pregnancy, regardless if men's spermatozoa met the egg or not. For the purpose of giving birth to a superman or a superwoman, the male presence is simply needed to awaken her dormant ability to procreate without the physical spermatozoa. It is very important that both man's and woman's body to be completely clean through chastity and raw food diet so that a genuine/ true parthenogenesis may occur.

Throughout time, it was not impossible that a parthenogenesis may have occurred, even if the bodies of the man and female were not clean, in that case the child would be no different than the rest of the world. In that case would have been a failed or not healthy parthenogenesis. The same as when a woman gets pregnant from precum (not mature spermatozoa) and from men's sperm who have ejaculated more than once within 74 days, which is the full maturity time of spermatozoa. Without intercourse, but with just loving and passionate kisses and hugs, a genuine parthenogenesis may occur ONLY when both sexes have been practicing chastity and a vegetarian diet (only raw fruit and vegetables).
– Liquid Metal

Some men may be offended or triggered by this subject. Do not feel inferior, neither men nor women are inferior to each other when both sexes fully honor their roles. There is a reason why men are build stronger, to build the physical world and make it a safe place for women. Some women may think they don't need protection from anyone. I advise you (both genders) to go beyond the surface way of thinking and feeling; observe nature, animals and reflect on everything. Go beyond what is deemed normal and moral in our society. When you do that, you will see that both men and women are equally important for a free and a peaceful society.

Neither extreme patriarchal, nor extreme matriarchal societies are good. Freedom, peace and prosperity for all is in the middle, where the union between the feminine and masculine meet. The dark powers/sorcerers have done the impossible to pin both sexes against each other. Women create life and they must be protected at all cost. Your children need a safe present and future. To achieve that, a clean body, mind and spirit is needed, otherwise man will see the woman as a piece of meat and woman will see man as someone to procreate and discard, like we see it in our modern society.

This corrupt system exists solely to control mankind, especially women which hold the portal to gain access to the physical world. This system, especially the education establishment, teaches how to maintain the status quo and to maximize shareholders' wealth at all cost, at the cost of people's blood (life energy).

Men build the physical world with their hands and strength, but women create the human temple, including men. So you see, how important the feminine is? Treat her like a Goddess so that she can give birth to Gods/sons and Goddesses/daughters. The woman harnesses the electromagnetic energy/astral forces of the 7 illuminaries and the 12 constellations so that the human body is manifested in the physical world.

If you still watch porn or driven by lust, you will have a hard time understanding some subjects in this book, especially this one. Since I stopped consuming dead flesh and other unnatural/unhygienic food and drinks; and stopped wasting my seed/sexual energy, I began to see the true reality of our existence. I don't see women as if they were beneath me, I don't see myself as being above them, I don't see them as piece of meat to use for sex. The moment you realize and practice this, is the moment you have begun the journey to becoming a superman or a super woman. You cannot fast for 3 days or a week and then after, you continue the same self-destructive lifestyle as before you fasted without damaging yourself. Which is better?:

1- Fast for two - three days once a month, and when you don't fast you consume alcohol, white refined flour and white refined sugar products, processed food and drinks, live in fear and worry, lying to yourself and others, waste your seminal fluids, conventional intercourse, masturbation?

2- Don't fast, eat daily but the meals are only fruit and vegetables, chaste life, honest to yourself and the world, caring about animals, not just dogs and cats but all animals.

Obviously, number 2 is the way to go. You've already read in this book how bad the body is affected by wasting the seminal fluid; and how bad it is when you consume all sorts of food and drinks that are deemed normal in our society. Fasting once in a while and at the same time you keep abusing your body with poison and toxic products, won't do much. Better to improve gradually a bit at a time, rather than making a big step (fasting) and then fall down again (going back to consuming toxic and unhygienic food and drinks).

Going back to 'Parthenogenesis', so what if a male's spermatozoa is not needed for the woman to procreate? Think about it, if you are a male, you won't have to waste your life force, which means that you will become intelligent, have high self esteem, you will become emotionally and mentally balanced, you will be very strong. Think with your upper head.

Many men and women detest the opposite gender because of some negative experiences of the past that they had. You must not condemn all men or all women just because you had a bad past relationship. The content of this book is about the superman/superwoman where both sexes equally respect and care/love one another, it is about going beyond this corrupt and decayed system of life. You cannot grasp the superman/superwoman concept if you stay in the current 3D mentality state. To understand what you don't understand, you must first question what you think you understand, you must question all beliefs you acquired all along until now.

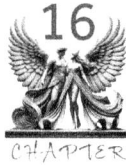

PREPARATIONS FOR AN IMMACULATE CONCEPTION

LET US NOW CONSIDER HOW A SUPERMAN CHILD may be immaculately conceived. First, its parents should not be under thirty-five years of age, the time when they reach full physical, mental and spiritual maturity. The reason why the ovum is not immaculately conceived when birth control methods are used is because there is not a sufficient strong electrical current than generated, which only exists when the vital fluid is conserved not only for several years before, but also during the act. For several years previous to conception, they should live in chastity, studying their mutual adaptability, and striving to make closer their inner soul-attunement. During this period they should both avoid physical and magnetic contact, so that their vital electricities might be at greatest intensity, and of the most opposite polarity, at the time of conception.

For an immaculate conception to be possible, a strong electrical attraction, or difference on potential, should exist between the parents; the greater their combined vitality, the more perfect will be the child. During this time, they should live in the country, preferably among the mountains, so that they may breathe in the pure, invigorating ozone, and be daily bathed by the vitalizing ultra-violet rays. They should subsist on a strict fruit diet.

Fruits are charged with higher solar vibration, containing radioactive energy which electrifies the body. This vitalization of the organism is greatly augmented by ultra-violet sun baths, which are necessary in preparation for an immaculate conception. Sunlight intensifies the body's vital magnetism, invigorates the ductless glands, electrifies the seminal fluid and enlivens the reproductive cells.

"New life and energy are brought about by a process which may be called a transmutation of electronic energy into physical and mental force. Redfield and Bright of Harvard Medical School found that seeds which had been exposed to the action of radium rays grew more rapidly than seeds not so treated. Hughes and Payne of Manhattan College, Kansas, found that hens exposed to ultraviolet rays laid four times as many eggs as the other hens. Professor Dawson Turner recently stated that by treating frog's eggs with radium he had bread frogs three times their normal size". – Bailey Radium Laboratories: Radithor

It must be remembered that an immaculate conception is not possible until the parents have, for at least a year, cured themselves of seminal emissions and menstruation, which may be accomplished by the fruit and nut diet, and by continent living. This conservation of vital fluid would sufficiently augment their electro-magnetic radiations to make an immaculate conception possible.

A menstruating woman has not sufficient vitality to conceive immaculately, nor a man subject to seminal emissions become the father of a superman. Therefore, the mothers of supermen were either barren, having not menstruated for many years previously (as in the case od Isaac, Jacob, Joseph, Samson, Samuel, Moses, Mary and John the Baptist), or virgins who have not yet commenced to menstruate (as in the case of Zoroaster and Jesus).

It was a custom among the Essenes, which was practiced prior to the birth of Mary, Jesus and John, that prospective parents should live in chastity and should know each other for at least three years before conception.

> *When parents live hygienically and continently, there will be no menopause or senility, and they will both be able to retain their reproductive capacities throughout their lives, which should be several centuries in length. While those who live in the poisonous atmosphere of the city, eating unnatural food, and depleting their vital forces by incontinence, have not enough magnetic power to conceive immaculately, those who lead this life among the mountains would be unable to do so.*

You are a walking miracle

And while two weak electric poles require a material conductor, between two strong ones, a current may be established directly through the ether. (*In this case the material conductor or conductors would be the egg and the spermatozoa, which are required for procreation when people's electrical poles are weak from consuming toxic products and wasting their life force i.e. semen/blood and eggs* – L.M).

By the initiative of the future mother, male and female magnetisms should, in a passionless and spiritual way, come into sufficient proximity to electrical impregnate and enliven the egg.

Professor Elmer Gates has demonstrated that evil emotions such as, fear, remorse or anger, create poisons in the blood which tend to retard or stop the growth of the cells of the body; while the good emotions such as, peace, joy, happiness, produce secretions which bring about a normal development of those cells. These secretions affect the reproductive cells, as well as the soma cells of the individual. Therefore, Professor Gates urges parents to put themselves in training and cherish only the right kind of emotions, the inspiring, high-grade feeling, for six months or a year before the initial of a new life takes place, in order that the productive cells may be perfectly formed and have in them the foundation for a strong, vigorous constitution in the offspring.

The month previous to conception should be one of special training, for at that time the ovum that is to be conceived is maturing, greatly increasing in size. The character of the human egg is entirely determined by the blood from which it is formed. The quality of this blood, in turn, is influenced by the varying physiological and psychological conditions of the mother, by her diet, and by her glandular secretions. The more hygienic her diet, and the longer her chastity previous to conception, the more vital will be the ovum, and the more physically, mentally and spiritually perfect will be the coming child. During this period of preparation (which should take place in a special Eugenic Community) prospective parents should concentrate their energies upon the cultivation of those talents which are to constitute the child's predetermined future life-work.

Commentary by **LIQUID METAL**

If you are already at an age where you can't have more children or you think it is too late to bring a super child in this world, don't feel bad, you didn't have information about this. Instead of feeling bad, teach your children the right information. And if you don't have children (and don't want to have any), then teach others so that their children will create a better world for everyone, including your grand children and any generation after that.

IS THERE ANOTHER WAY TO CREATE A SUPER CHILD?

To create a superchild, there may be another way, and that is very difficult. That would be white tantric sex, sexual intercourse between two people that fully circulate their energy/life force between them, where the battery effect is completed. But the man must not ejaculate at all, the same applies for the woman (she must also not menstruate). He and she should have been chaste for a few years prior. And of course, both the woman and the man must have been on a raw food diet for a long time.

I wouldn't advise this method, because it is very difficult to not ejaculate while having sexual intercourse. Being able to not ejaculate is only half of the method, the other half is raising the energy and the life force upward your spine while conscious. It has to be equal for both the man and the woman.

So, the method/lifestyle (vegetarian diet and chastity) mentioned in this book is the easier way. They are both difficult methods if you don't think is possible or if you have a hard time letting go of sex (orgasm, masturbation, arousal), if you have a hard time letting go of all food except fruit and vegetables. While on vegetarian diet, I almost fell a few times, I was about to consume bread, and cooked food since I live in the same house with people that consume products other than fruit and vegetables.

It takes determination and discipline to become the ONE. Anyone that you know, who gets sick or dies; those situations are opportunities for you to stop abusing your body. Life throws hints at you daily; you got to listen to the subtle or not so subtle messages that whisper at you all the time. You can learn from other people's mistakes.

But being on a fruit diet is much better, it is the next higher step from fruit-vegetable diet. The information in this book may be beyond of what you are capable right now, but take one step at a time. Knowledge is a gift; knowledge must not be hoarded but shared with others. Share this knowledge with others, some may be stronger than us, so by sharing knowledge, we help ourselves regardless. One day perhaps our children will get together with the children of those parents we shared the knowledge with.

DON'T LIE TO YOURSELF

Most of us lie to ourselves. We think we are healthy; we think our children are the best children. Lies, lies, and more lies. Do you ever get mad, worried, anxious etc.? All of us do at one point or another, which that means that we are not healthy. Just being able to walk, munch on food and breathe, doesn't make us healthy. Most people think they are healthy, but if they did a thorough examination of themselves, they would realize that they are dying, they are marching toward the grave one step at a time.

Somewhere here I mentioned that neither a patriarchal nor matriarchal system is good. We know that a predominant patriarchal system will try and suppress women, there will be wars for all kinds of reasons, including wars over imaginary gods in the sky. A matriarchal only system might seem good on the surface, there won't be wars because women are nurturers, they will nurture children for peace. But what you may not know is that according to the natural order of creation, there is a full 25.900 years of natural cycle (12 zodiac ages).

There are ebb and flow constantly, there are Golden and Silver but also Bronze and Iron/Dark ages where humanity lives in darkness and ignorance. No matter how peaceful a society will be, a time comes where it changes, where feminine gets captured. I do not know if this is by universal design to ensure survival of creation where things balance themselves out, or whether there are higher beings out there that have created this system for us in this reality, to keep us going in circles.

That's why it is important that we create a society of both men and women where unity prevails. You got to go beyond the normal way of thinking. Feel the truth from within. What you eat and drink affect your intuition where you may lose the path to enlightenment.

Don't forget that this information of how to conceive a superman, is not simply for the purpose of giving birth to a child. Even if you don't want to have children, by following a strict raw food diet and chastity, you become immortal and you will retain all the memories and experiences of this lifetime so that when you reincarnate again, assuming you'd want to, you will be born will all the memories intact. You won't have to redo again a 3D reality/school of struggling and suffering from amnesia.

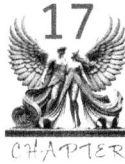

THE PSYCHOLOGY OF CONCEPTION

THE PHILOSOPHERS HOLD THAT TO ENGENDER CHILDREN is the most sacred and filial duty of man. Both man and woman are taught by them that the aim and aspiration of union is to enter into a conscious relationship with the incoming ego or soul. Their disciples seek so to prepare and govern themselves that they may be worthy to bring a soul manifesting in the loftiest and purest levels of consciousness into incarnation on earth, thereby giving life to a more highly evolved being than is possible for unthinking minds, impure hearts and unprepared bodies to attract.

The Philosopher, being in conscious relationship with the incoming ego, affords it great assistance as it passes through the denser states of matter, and encourages it to incarnate or enter the physical body prior to birth; for then for a time it cringes from assuming its dense physical vestment, since, as it were, it dies to the world from which it came. Through knowledge of Nature's Law and obedience to it, the Philosopher has power to attract from the Heavenly World those perfected beings who come as messengers to the race.

"Purity of body, mind and soul, and the worship of God through the being beloved, ever bring into life on earth a soul beautified by its own Divine Source. And if two people, having physical characteristics which are ugly, worship God through the being beloved, with purity of mind and heart, the law of hereditary physical resemblance will be modified and the offspring will radiate that which is of the soul.

The child which is a product of unpurified, ungoverned and

unhallowed passion and desire becomes the vehicle of an ego of like character but more dominant in will, with inclinations equalling the sum of the passions and desires of the unthinking parents. Such are in truth the children of wrath and malediction for whose salvation the Philosophers, through reverent preparation of body, soul and spirit for parenthood, seek to bring into incarnation those beings who are chosen vessels of the Divine Love and Wisdom". – Monfaucon: *Comte de Gabalis*

("To me, God is Nature, the whole creation, the Void or whatever it is that holds everything together. To me God is not a person. It is fine if you think it is a person, as long as what you do, contributes to the raising of your consciousness and in the betterment of the world, as long as you are your own authority in life, by honoring creation and obeying the Natural Law/ Laws". – Liquid Metal)

The thoughts and feelings of the parents at the moment of conception will determine the kind of soul they will attract, and the future destiny of the child. Pliny said:

"It is believed that whatever is seen, heard, remembered, or thought of, at the time of conception is very potent in causing resemblance".

In the Bible, we find the following example of the operation of this law:

"Jacob took him rods of green poplar; and of the hazel and chestnut tree; and pilled white streaks in them, and made the white appear which was in the rods. And he set the rods which he had pilled before the flocks in the gutters in the watering troughs when the flocks came to drink, that they should conceive when they came to drink. And the flocks conceived before the rods, and brought forth cattle ring-streaked, speckled and spotted".

Alexander the Great's conception took place in a temple called "The House of Gods". At that time, his mother spiritually saw a divine being coming to her, inspiring her with the thought that her child would be a future world-leader. - "Message of the Stars" by Max Heindel

---

Conception should be preceded by prayer and meditation, and by inward communion of the parents with the unborn soul they are to receive upon Earth. There should be special Eugenic Temples for this purpose. The hearing of elevating music previous to, and even during conception is very beneficial; also the visualization and beholding of the forms of ideal human beings.

Best of all would be to have such an individual actually present - for then there will be a spiritual as well as a visual impression. **Conception should not take place in a city, or in a mundane dwelling place**, but in a Eugenic Sun-Temple, situated, as is an astronomical observatory, on the top of a lofty mountain, in an ethereal and ultra-violet atmosphere. When thus performed, in the presence of a Eugenic Educator, there would be no shame, passion or emotion attached to the act, but only a holy feeling of service to humanity and devotion to the unborn soul.

Marriage was instituted by the angels as a sacrament, and the sacred rite of generation was performed under the supervision in great temples at certain times of the year when interplanetary lines of force were propitious for propagation. The rest of the time all lived together in a paradisiacal bliss of chaste companionship. Therefore parturition was painless, and sickness and sorrow were unknown.

Conception should never take place at night, nor when either parents is not at the height of his of her physical, mental and spiritual vitality. Man, like woman, has a monthly magnetic rhythm, a periodic increase and decrease of vitality. Since this commences at birth, it occurs at different times for different people. However, the chaste association of the prospective parents during the period of preparation would result in the equalization of their magnetic rhythms, so that these would finally occur simultaneously. At a certain day of the lunar month (ordinarily directly after the menstrual period) their combined vitality should be at its point of maximum intensity, which is the proper time (in the monthly cycle) for conception.

There is a similar increase and decrease of vitality every twenty-four hours, which fixes, for each pair of parents, a certain hour of the day best suited for conception. Usually, this would be in the late afternoon, when terrestrial, physiological and solar currents are at greatest intensity. Conception should take place in the ultra-violet sunshine, amidst the soothing green color of nature, and in an atmosphere of peace, harmony and holiness, if the best possible results are desired.

There is also a certain zodiacal month in the solar cycle best adapted for the conception of each child, according to its predetermined life-work, which may be astrologically computed.

Thus, the month, day and hour for conception may, and should be decided upon beforehand. Conception should not take place without eugenic sanction, after at least a year's preparatory training.

Krishna and Buddha were conceived in a forest. The newly married parents of Pythagoras were sent by the Delphic Oracle to a distant country so that the predestined son might be conceived, formed and born far from the disturbing influence of his own land.

Commentary by LIQUID METAL

ARE YOU POSSESSED?

What do you think when you read or think about the term "being possessed"? Chances are you'd think about movies such as "The Exorcist". Of course, that movie is exaggerated, even though in some cases, there may be people being possessed like that. But the real possession is our world. Most people are walking zombies (The Walking Dead Tv show is a metaphor for the masses). Most people are possessed.

If you drink alcohol (spirit suppressor), you are possessed.
If you consume meat (dead flesh full of parasites) you are possessed.
If you ejaculate (or have sexual intercourse), you are possessed.
If you lie and deceive, you are possessed.
If you consume sugar, processed food and drinks, you are possessed.
If you are worried or scared in anyway, you are possessed.
If you gossip, if you are greedy for money and materialistic objects you are possessed.
If you believe and trust any authority except your own, you are possessed.

All the above are normal in our society. Calling all these, 'possessions', in the eyes of the masses, would make me look like a lunatic, or a crazy person. Am I? It takes a real sharp thinking to truly analyze ourselves on a deeper level. This Earth is a mental asylum, the bars of the prison are invisible, they are mental.

OBEY THE NATURAL LAW

The true meaning of "obedience to God" is to obey the Natural Law/Laws of Nature. If you don't, you will decay, die and keep reincarnating in 3D reality. But the organized religion, through devious tactics, conditions people to believe that God is an actual physical person. You are created based on the Natural Law, without it, you could not be born. There are different layers, for example, if you were conceived through sexual intercourse, your parents did not obey the Natural Law, therefore you were born incomplete, meaning already began to die the moment you were born. Obeying to the Natural LAW means to not ingest filth in your body and mind and to not procreate through the animalistic, lower consciousness method of procreation which is "physical sexual intercourse".

THE MOMENT OF CONCEPTION ATTRACTS LIFE OR DEATH

The physical, emotional and mental state you are at the moment of conception, will attract a healthy or a sick spirit. You could think that sickness exists only in a physical body. Where do you think your soul is, 50km away from you? Your soul is where you are right now, at all times, except for when you sleep, your soul may wonder around in different realms, but always attached with a silver cord to the physical body. The moment the cord is cut/detached, then the body cannot be alive anymore.

People have one night stands, or have sexual intercourse while under alcohol influence or when their body is filthy, filled of toxicity from food and drinks. And on top of that, most people's physical vessel is depleted of their lifeforce from indulging in sexual activities. What these do, is that you attract spirits of the same quality that your vessel is. When someone's physical vessel/body expires, meaning when they die, if that person was an alcoholic, or anything else that polluted their body and the mind while alive, their spirit will be confused and attached to the earthly habits.

The spirits wander in the astral realm for an exit. Just as if you were in the forest wandering confused and panicked to find the path home, so is the polluted spirit. The moment of conception will attract a spirit that is of the same quality of the future parents of the child at that moment.

Sometimes, in our lives we see very good parents but not so good children and vice versa. First of all, we see others as we are, and secondly, we don't know if the good parents/people are actually good. Most people are fake, most people lie to themselves daily, most people keep secrets, resentments, hate and grudge inside of themselves, so the outside world/people think they know them but that is not true at all. Having in mind also the karmic debts (assuming you believe there is such a thing), sometimes some bad spirits may incarnate in great and loving parents and vice versa.

Based on their previous life, perhaps in this life they will have to deal with a bad child and vice versa. So that I don't overwhelm you any more than it is needed, cut the problem from the root which is to not consume anymore toxic food, drinks, thoughts/information. Otherwise, the parents' soul and the future/newborn's soul together is very powerful, in a negative or in a positive way, depending on the quality of the parents. So, technically, the parents invite the lost and unpurified spirit to enter their child's life/body, unknowingly to the parents on a conscious level.

But do not think that a child is condemned forever as a result of ignorant conception. Every moment of the day you have the free will and power to choose any path you wish. A good or a bad path. Every day you can choose health or disease. Nothing is incurable.

When   Nicolas Pierre Henri de Monfaucon in *Comte De Gabalis* mentioned about beings being chosen vessels of the Divine Love and Wisdom, don't think that others choose whom lives and who dies. You too can be the chosen one. As I previously mentioned, you decide how your life turns out to be, or how you children's or grandchildren's life turns out to be. Let it begin with you, when you practice raw food diet (the ultimate goal being "Breatharianism") and chastity, then you are planting the seeds so that your child is chosen, then his child will be chosen and so on.

If we are too weak to let go of all the poisons that this system produces, then we will decay and repeat the same life (under different characters) over and over again until we get it right. By the way, your own choices dictate your physical body's expiration date or not expiry at all. Do not fall for "aging and death are normal", they are not normal. The word "normal" is very dangerous. Anything repeated enough it gets normalized. Normalize health, love and care and not the opposites.

PART V

PRENATAL CULTURE

"Before I formed thee in the belly I knew thee; and before thou camest forth out of the womb I sanctified thee, and I ordained thee a prophet unto the nations". – Jeremiah

"Parents alone benefit their children prior to their birth, and are the cause to their offspring of all their upright conduct". – Pythagoras

PRENATAL INFLUENCE

DR. H. W. LONG, A PHYSICIAN, PSYCHOANALYST AND NEUROLOGIST, after subjecting the problem of prenatal influence to a scientific investigation, has come to the conclusion that it is a reality. In his book, "Motherhood", he cites a large number of cases which have come under his observation, showing a definite co-relation between the mother's psychological condition during gestation and the character of the resulting child. Many great men have owed their talent to prenatal influence. Napoleon's case is described by Dr. Long as follows:

"**Napoleon**'s mother is considered by some students of history to be even more remarkable than her famous son. During this gestation, she accompanied her husband on a military campaign, becoming acquainted with many of the officers, had the walls of her room hung with paintings of many famous generals, and was deeply interested in all military matters. It has been said that she had her accouchement couch covered with a tapestry depicting one of the battles of Thermopylae".

Van Dyck's mother was a talented artist. She was diligently engaged in the work which she regarded as her masterpiece, while pregnant with the child who was to make her famous in the history of art. It was a large composition in colored silk entitles "Susanna and the Elders".

During **Goethe**'s gestation, his mother, under her husband's instruction, devoted her time to study. Goethe inherited his poetic and imaginative temperament from her.

Schopenhauer's mother, during her entire period of pregnancy, lived alone in a country villa, in whose library she cultivated her literary tastes.

Charles Kingsley acquired his talents from his mother. In faith that the impressions made on her own mind before the birth of the child for whose coming she longed, would be mysteriously transmitted to him. Mrs. Kingsley luxuriated in the romantic surrounding of her Devonshire home, and gave herself up every sight and sound which she hoped would be dear to her child in afterlife. Her hopes, we know, were fully realized.

Samson's mother, in accordance with an angel's command, abstained from the use of wine and meat during gestation. She held in her mind the thought of her son's future life work, that he would lead his people against the Philistines.

Buddha was afforded exceptionally favourable prenatal conditions. The king rejoiced exceedingly, and gave orders that all care might be taken of his queen during her pregnancy; that wherever she might be, she might be surrounded by that which was pure, melodious, harmonious, refined, elegant and simple.

The mother of **Confucius**, before the birth of her child, heard a heavenly voice predict his destiny: "*The son of the essence of water shall succeed the decaying Chou, and be a throneless king*".

During **Alexander the Great**'s gestation, his mother lived in a temple, in the company of a great Egyptian philosopher.

Concerning the prenatal history of **Apollonius of Tyana**, we read: "During the period which preceded his birth, his mother was favoured with a kind of annunciation sent by the god of divination and penetrative science. **Proteus** appeared to her, and informed her that the child of whom she was pregnant was an incarnation of himself".

The following is recorded concerning the mother of **St. David of Wales**:

"As her womb was growing, the mother, for the purpose of offering alms and oblations for childbirth according to current customs, enters a certain church, to hear the preaching of the gospel. Gildas, the preacher, says: "'The son, who is in the womb of that nun has grace and power and rank greater than I, because God has given him status and sole rule and primacy over all the saints of Brittania forever. One thing was clearly manifest to all, that she was to bring forth into the world one who is honourable status, effulgent wisdom, and eloquent speech would excel all the doctors of Brittania"

Before the birth of Thomas Aquinus, a rough hermit with flowing hair, like Elias, who gained a name for his godly life pointed to a picture of St. Dominic which hung from an image of Blessed Virgin around his neck, and exclaimed: "Rejoice, O lady, for though art with child, and thou shalt bring forth a son, whom thou shalt call Thomas; and thou and thy husband shall make a monk of him". A similar man came too the pregnant mother of St. Francis, predicting her child's destiny.

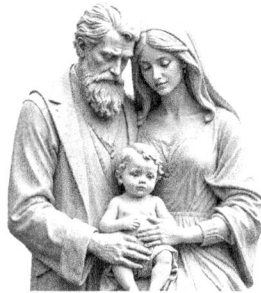

Prenatal influence is effected through the maternal blood. Since the embryo is a condensation of elements derived from this blood, the chemical quality of the latter will influence the development of the unborn child. The factor which may most immediately effect the blood's chemistry is the mother's diet. If the mother's blood is toxic, as a result of the use of drugs, alcohol or tobacco, the resulting child will be physically and mentally subnormal. Dr. Tilney, the neurologist, in speaking concerning his proposed research work along this line, said:

"We shall be able to determine departures from the normal standard in children whose mother has suffered from some poisoning prior to childbirth. Such poisoning may be due to alcohol, tobacco, bromides or veronal. The next step will be to determine whether this deviation is sufficient to retard the mental development of the child. We might discover that tobacco or alcohol produces a mild deviation from the normal, and that a certain dietary deficiency in the expectant mother or an injury to her liver is responsible for maladjustment in a child which results in a savage or unsocial outlook on life".

On the other hand, great purity of the mother's blood, as occurs when no meat or wine is used during gestation, will lead to the birth of a superior child. The mothers of Chrishna, Samson, Buddha, Jesus, St. David and Honen Shonin lived upon a vegetarian diet during gestation. The blood passing from the mother to the child contains internal secretions, chemically representing all organs of her body, and reproducing these, in miniature form, in the embryo. Between the ductless glands of the mother and the organs of the embryo there is even closer relationship than between these glands and the mother's own organs.

These glandular secretions (which are greatly influenced by the organic minerals in the diet and by impulses from the central nervous system, registering psychological states) profoundly affect embryonic development. **A weakened or sickly condition of any member of the mother's body** (due to a glandular and dietetic cause) **will result in an improper development of a corresponding organ in the embryo**. And inversely, an exercising and strengthening of any maternal organ, accompanied by an increase secretion of associated ductless glands, will enhance the growth of a corresponding embryonic organ.

This relationship (prenatal influence) takes place directly through the blood. Physical and psychological traits are inherited in this way, rather than through the germ-cell. Inheritance of paternal traits, as in the case of the Bach family, is due to the prenatal impression by the mother of the qualities the father manifested during gestation.

There is an interdependent relationship between the ductless glands and the organs they control. The thyroids, for instance, are associated with cerebral activity; and the exercise of those maternal brain-centers which these glands control, will, through the influence of their hormones, augment the growth of similar centers in the embryo. As there is a relationship (through the blood) between the bodily organs of mother and child, so is there one between the respective parts of the brain. The thoughts, images, perceptions, aspirations and ideals in the mind of the expectant mother will, in this way, materialize themselves as potential cerebral faculties in the embryo.

Emotional states, because of the different glandular secretions by which they are accompanied, may affect, for good or ill, embryonic development. These glandular secretions, produced by thoughts and emotions, will activate the growth of similar ductless glands and brain centers in the embryo, thereby laying in the child the physiological basis for the reappearance of the psychological faculties which the mother has exercised during gestation.

The phenomenon of protective coloration illustrates the capacity of an organism to reproduce on the surface of its skin that which its senses perceive. Stigmatization and hypnotic suggestibility demonstrate that the human body possesses similar capacities. If the perception, mental images, emotions and thoughts of a woman are able to affect the cells of her own body, even those of peripheral regions, surely they must have a far greater influence upon the plastic substance of the embryo. That we do not as yet know the exact physiological mechanism by which this is accomplished does not invalidate the reality of the phenomenon.

Potential genius, along an line, may be insured in the coming child if the pregnant mother concentrates upon the cultivation of these abilities, especially when these express her own natural endowments. Dr. Long says: "By and by, parents will come to understand that by giving special attention to any faculty or quality they desire to have reproduced in their offspring, they can have their wished gratified just in proportion to the intelligent effort expended.

The following is a typical case recorded by Dr. Long:
"Case 136: Mrs. W. is somewhat musical in her tastes, as is also her husband, and when she found herself pregnant, they began together a systematic study and practice of music. They enjoyed the work, attending all the concerts possible, and frequently went to dances where they might hope to hear good music. The son resulting from this gestation began very early to show a taste and talent for music, both vocal and instrumental. His cleverness and skill were so marked that he was considered a prodigy by many who heard him, and is now a professional musician of high standing".

Riddell, in "Prenatal Culture", reports the following case:

"A man who came from an inventive family, who was not a mechanic, undertook to produce a mechanical invention, and worked on it prior to the birth of his son. During gestation the mother became much interested in the invention and entered heavily into the study with him. The boy born under these circumstances began his inventions before the age of ten.

At twenty-five he had produced over 20 original inventions and double as many improvements, several of which paid well. That this inventive genius and originality of mind were largely the result of prenatal training is proven by the fact that the older children show very little mechanical ingenuity and scarcely a trace of originality, while children born after the inventive son showed more incentive talent than the older one but have not the inventive power of the one who received the special prenatal training".

The varied characteristics of children born from the same parents and raised in the same environments can only be explained by the prenatal theory of heredity, not by the germ-cell one. Children born from the same father, but from different mothers, as illustrated by the children of Abraham and by those of the father of Daniel Webster, who had children by two different wives, always take after their respective mothers.

Not only the father's psychological traits, but also his physical traits, are transmitted to the child through prenatal influence, rather than through the germ-cell. Where parents were separated during gestation, as were those of Leonardo da Vinci, Schopenhauer and Oscar Wilde, there was little paternal resemblance. The father is usually the mother's prenatal model whose image is implanted upon the embryo. Dr. Long says: "In Italy it has been observed that many of the children resemble the pictures and statues of the child Jesus, as a result of the mother's adoration of the Madonna. The Weismannian germ-cell theory, though applicable to animal reproduction, cannot explain the phenomena of human inheritance.

Commentary by **LIQUID METAL**

Remember when Proteus said that he was an incarnation of himself? That was a situation of beings that each previous life was better than the next. Meaning that they obeyed the Natural Laws, they didn't abuse their bodies. They lived a chaste life. Their life force was not extinguished like most people's is. When you life force is intact, when your consciousness level is high, you decide in which parents to reincarnate next. But, if you live a mundane, boring and uncareful life where you are selfish and abuse your body, then when you pass away, you will be so confused that you will reincarnate in a family where your life will be difficult or boring/mundane.

The only major mistake of any parent is to have had children that were conceived through the ordinary (sexual intercourse) way of procreating. I'm just as guilty as any parent. But we cannot go back in time, what we can do it to improve and progress from now on. You may be a parent that love your children and would disagree when I said about procreating through sexual intercourse is a major mistake. The truth (*how a real true powerful and healthy male or female should be conceived*) doesn't care what we think, what we feel and what we believe. Only lies need to defend themselves.

That you love your children is normal, everyone should love their offsprings. I will remind you again, do not forget what this book is about, it's about conceiving a superman or a superwoman, meaning fully healthy and immortal, and if you don't want to conceive again, then the information in this book applies just the same, if you just want to achieve a very long life or immortality without having to multiply yourself any further.

In general, in our demoralized society, many people are purposeless, lazy and defeated mentally, emotionally and spiritually. I hear sometimes people saying: "We will die anyway, so what's the point?". Throughout my life I have heard the same people change their tune when they got sick, or when someone they knew, passed away. Intelligence is when you consciously do something about your health and not as an after effect/reactionary when it might be too late by then.

Even though this book talks about having to let go everything that we deem normal (sex, sugar, salt, cooked food, alcohol, coffee etc.), use it as fuel to improve your life. Let go of one thing at a time. Whether you are a woman or a man, it doesn't matter. What matters is to purify your blood which nourishes all your organs, including the brain. Each step that you consciously take, will lead you to greatness.

If you want your children to develop or be born with talents, then you should practice those talents while in gestation period, and even better if you begin practicing even before conceiving. Even if you think you are not capable of playing a musical instrument, then listen to instrumental music while the child is conceived, or any other talents you wish him or her to have. Humans may only have ears on their head, but all the cells of the body are constantly listening to your words and thoughts which result in action.

There is no reason to be bored in life, if boredom arrives, then change must happen. Excite yourself with newness. Walk or drive in a different route than usual, go somewhere where you've never been before. It doesn't have to be a different country, it can be a different place within the same country, as long as it is a happy place, meaning NATURE. It is sad to feel bored in this beautiful land.

I don't really watch movies, but when I do, I watch movies that have a meaning, that empowers me to be appreciative of what I have. I was watching "Water World" a 1995 movie, it was about a postapocalyptic world where there was no land, everywhere there was water for much of their lives, or so they thought. Eventually, some of the characters through a lot of struggling and emotional rollercoasters, found lush green land. They were so happy to see dry land as if that was the best thing in their lives. And yet, we have been living on dry land since birth and we complain. In life, when you lose something, you appreciate it more.

Don't fall for "happiness is out there", happiness is where you are at any given moment. Let go of the weight (ungratefulness, unappreciation, complaining, gossiping, resentment, worries, fears, fear of old age, fear of dying, trying to be someone who you are not, lying to yourself and others etc.) and all you'll be left with, is, "happiness".

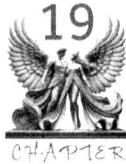

THE INFLUENCE OF MATERNAL CHASTITY UPON THE BRAIN DEVELOPMENT OF THE EMBRYO

THE EMBRYO IS A CONDENSATION OF THE MATERNAL BLOOD; and for an embryonic superman to be formed, super-blood is required. The blood of the mother is enriched and vitalized chiefly by her glandular secretions, particularly by those of the sex glands. There exists a very intimate relationship between the maternal genital secretions, or hormones, and the growing brain of the fetus. On this account, excessive sexual intercourse, previous to conception and during gestation, by draining the mother's blood of genital secretions which are otherwise lymphatically absorbed and used for the construction of embryonic brain-tissue (since these secretions are very rich in phosphorus, the principal element required for the formation of nerve-cells), results in the birth of a physically and mentally subnormal child.

"Many ills and great suffering are directly traceable to excessive sexual intercourse during the non-pregnant state; and sexual intercourse during pregnancy is responsible for an almost endless list of physical and mental defects, ranging all the way from color-blindless to idiocy; and the number of physical and mental defectiveness, due to this cause, is rapidly increasing from year to year. It is also responsible for universal unhappiness among married women who know instinctively that it is harmful". - Thurston: *Thurston's Philosophy of Marriage*

Maternal chastity, before and after conception, leads to opposite results.

Eames, in "The Principle of Eugenics" describes an experiment in which the reproductive cells of an individual were microscopically examined after a period of dissipation, and again, after one of continence. In the latter case they were larger and more vital than in the former. The author remarks that children born from devitalized reproductive cells would be physically and mentally inferior to those born from the others.

Therefore, the superman of the past were born either from young virgins or from mothers of advanced age who were considered barren. In both cases they were women who were not menstruating. There is an important reason for this – for **menstruating involves a periodic loss of seminal fluid, thereby draining the blood of elements required for a superior embryonic brain**. For a superman to be born, it is therefore necessary that his mother be non-menstruating virgin. The longer the genital fluid of the mother is preserved within her body previous to conception, the superior (physically, mentally and spiritually) will be the coming child.

All great men had pious and chaste mothers (though their fathers were not always so), as were those of Zoroaster, Krishna, Samuel, Buddha, Plato, Confucius, Mary, John te Baptist, Jesus, St. Agustine, St. Bernard, St. Francis, Thomas Aquinus, St. Theresa, George Fox, Wesley, Rembrandt, Beethoven, Priestley, Locke, Kant, Pestalozzi, Abraham Lincoln, Mary Baker Eddy and Annie Besant. In an ancient writing, it is stated that the unborn Buddha reflected on her who should be his mother.

According to the customs of Buddha, he could not be born of any ill-conducted, immoral person, but of one who had passed stainlessly through countless generations, and had never offended against the Five Great Commandments, abstinence from:

1- **the eating of animal food**
2- **stealing**
3- **sexual indulgence**
4- **untruthfulness**
5- **the drinking of alcoholics**

There are important physiological reasons why continence during the period preceding conception (involving not only abstinence from sexual activity but also the complete conservation of genital fluid) is necessary if a superior child is to be produced. The human egg – at the commencement of its development, is much like a hen's egg – containing white germinal substance and a yolk in the center. The chemical composition of this yolk (the first external material to enter into the embryonic brain) is determined by the blood supply to the ovaries during the period previous to conception. Any loss of genital fluid during that time impoverishes and devitalizes the blood, and deprives the yolk of the maturing ovum of the phosphorus compound required for the nourishment of the embryo's brain-tissues, at the commencement of its development.

Before Alexander the Great's conception, his mother lived alone in a temple. Mary's parents, previous to her conception, lived for about twenty years, chastely. St. Patrick was born from parents who lived in chastity both before and after his conception. His father was a priest; and it was then the rule that clergymen were permitted to marry if they lived chastely with their wives. St. David was born of a nun, who neither before nor after (his conception) knew a man, but, continuing in chastity of mind and body, led a most faithful life.

Isaac Newton's father died before his birth, his mother not marrying until three years later. Not only were conditions after his conception comparatively chaste, but also those before. It is stated upon good authority that Sir Isaac Newton was conceived after two years of enforced continence. The exemplary life, spotless chastity and towering genius of the eminent philosopher testify to his splendid inheritance. Many are indebted to a life cause for their superior qualities. Nietzsche was his mother's first child, born four years after marriage. Since his father was a minister, we may assume comparatively chaste conditions prior to his birth.

Continence during gestation, which is universally practiced by healthy animals, unperverted primitive people and Indians (I'm assuming Dr. Raymond meant the Natives which falsely were called Indians, and not the Indians of the country India – T.M), is a law of nature. After its fertilization, the egg attaches itself to the uterine mucous membranes, which then thicken and swell, so that their glands may produce increased secretions for the nourishment of the embryo. These glandular secretions fill the cavity of the uterus, in which the embryo is developing, its cervical opening being plugged by sticky mucous, so that all of this valuable fluid may be retained.

The first differentiation to appear on the embryo is the neural canal, the beginning of the spine, brain and nervous system. The young embryo is almost all brain-tissue. At the end of the first month of its development, when it is half an inch in length, its head is larger than the rest of the body.

The younger the brain, the more plastic and sensitive it is, and the more durable are impressions made upon it. During its early formation, the size and chemical quality of the embryonic brain are largely determined by the character of its nutrition (by certain organic minerals, such as phosphorus, which are obtained from the secretions of the genital glands). The embryo is nourished first by the yolk-sac attached to it; then by the glandular secretions in the uterus, and finally by the maternal blood, conveyed to it through the placenta and the umbilical cord.

The uterine secretions are then absorbed by lymphatics and transmitted to the embryo through the blood. The quality of these secretions is determined by the mother's diet, and by the degree ti which they are conserved within the body through chastity. Intercourse through pregnancy, by causing coincident and subsequent discharges (by orgasm and by leucorrhea) of these secretions, the raw material of embryonic brain-tissue interferes with and retards the normal development of the unborn child.

The violation of natural law (any sex relationships from conception until childbirth) leads to the following **SEVEN** serious consequences:

ONE - Miscarriage or still birth.

TWO - The various sicknesses of pregnancy, such as morning sickness and nausea. (Continence, combined with proper diet, makes pregnancy a period of increased health, without the disorders which usually accompany it).

THREE - Nervous disturbances, such as neurasthenia and hysteria.

FOUR - Haemorrhages during parturition, puerperal fever, and death of mother or child during or after childbirth.

FIVE - By causing the escape from the uterus of glandular secretions which are normally absorbed and used for the nourishment and invigoration of the brain and nervous system of mother and child, it not only causes neurasthenic and hysterical symptoms in her, but leads to the birth of nervous and idiotic children.

SIX - It results in a mechanical and chemical irritation of the female genital tract, introducing into it extraneous matter which settles on the surface of the embryo, appearing as the "vernix caseosa", the foul smelling, cheesy substance which covers the newborn child. This substance decomposes, generating poisonous toxins which interfere with normal embryonic development, causing feeble-mindedness, color blindless, blindness and skin disease. The effect of the male seminal fluid upon the embryo is particularly injurious when it is poisoned by the use of tobacco or alcohol. By lymphatic absorption, the organism of the mother is also injured.

Dr. P. T. Johnson, an Indian physician, said: "Our people have always known, and the old mothers of the tribe teach, that sexual connection after pregnancy is the cause of the condition known to the medical profession as 'vernix caseosa', and they forbid intercourse during that time. Skin diseases are unknown among primitive people, nor are they afflicted with sore or weak eyes".

Dr. E. B. Marchall says: "The Dunkards refrain from sex relations during pregnancy, and I do remember a single case where there was an appreciable amount of vernix caseosa on an infant born of a Dunkard during my long practice of twenty-five years among these people".

Dr. Hubbard states: "I have kept a record of more than a hundred cases and have found that in every case, where there had been no sex congress after pregnancy had set in, that the child was born free from that unctuous substance, vernix caseosa; but where sex relation existed, the child was covered with more or less of this poisonous substance".

Rr. Hilscher says: "Reliable statistics are given in which it is stated that one-third of the blind in Europe become so from the poison of vernix, and that alone".

Male seminal fluids inside the mother while in pregnancy, implants morbid erotic impulses in the child (such as the tendency to masturbate). This is due to prenatal influence, but more particularly to the effect of the lymphatically absorbed male seminal fluid.

SEVEN – It causes difficult and painful childbirth.
Intercourse during pregnancy, frequently causes an interruption of the gestation (miscarriage), and occasionally puerperal sepsis (blood poisoning). It also causes a terrific excitation on the part of the mother, which is transmitted to and injures the unborn child, causing it to be less near to perfection in physique and mentality than was intended by Nature, and than it would have been had the mother been left alone by the male during pregnancy to develop the child properly.

If a virile bull breaks into a pen with a pregnant cow, the latter will make every effort within her power to avoid him. If she be unable to do so, the stock raiser always expects to be presented later on with a defective calf. This calf may have three or five legs, or two tails or two heads, or an abnormal number of internal organs, or it may have minor defects not readily noticeable; and this principle applies to the breeding of all other animals, including human beings. When an accident of this kind occurs, the stock raiser does not attempt to attribute it to any other than its true cause, i.e., sexual intercourse during pregnancy; and his natural procedure is to make better provision for the future to keep bulls away from his pregnant cows.

Human beings, in the belief that they are immune from the consequences of violating the natural laws which govern the relationship of the sexes among animals, use present marriage laws as an excuse for forcing a woman in pregnancy and out, to occupy the same bed or habitation with a man who is in fact, only a bull in human form, in so far as sex matters are concerned. The belief that a man cannot go for long periods without sexual intercourse is everywhere current. This is only true if he be subjected nightly to terrific sex appeal of a semi-nude bed companion. As this condition universally prevails, it results in the universal indulgence of an unbridled sexual passion.

Among the lower animals, the female selects the male most pleasing to her, unhampered in her choice by any latent desire for food, clothing or protection. She then permits the male so selected to have sexual intercourse with her, until she is pregnant, then, in certain species, she either drives him away, or leaves him. In others, she permits him to remain nearby to help provide for the young, but she does not, in the natural state outside of captivity, allow the male to have sexual intercourse with her again, until a certain time after the birth of the offspring.

Compare this eminently sensible conduct of the lower animal with present customs and teachings of human beings throughout the greater portion of the world that lead young girls to believe that sexual intercourse is improper until marriage, and imply that any amount of it after marriage is natural, legal and proper. Such customs and teachings are almost wholly responsible for the millions of the disillusioned, diseased, unhappy, embittered married and ex-married men and women now living, and also for hordes of unwanted, defective, unhappy children, who fill the slums of every city, and who are to be found in lesser numbers in every community throughout the world.

The majority of physicians now practicing have been taught that sexual intercourse during pregnancy is allowable up to the eighth month; and many of these physicians have been passing this information on to their women patients for years. Many of these physicians now realize that the practice is harmful and that they may have been indirectly responsible for scores of miscarriages, with their frequently resultant injurious complications, and for many defective children.

Frequently, however, an obstetrician will be found who will state in unqualified terms that sexual intercourse during pregnancy is horrible; that it is positively injurious to both mother and child, and that it places human beings on a moral plane below that of the lower animals.

"When all women learn the potential value of their possession, and also learn the vital necessity of its conservation after marriage as well as before, then the species will become magnificent in strength of body and brilliance of mind; radiant health will make it immune to disease, life will be indefinitely prolonged; revolutionary achievements by both men and women will follow each other in rapid succession". – Thurston, *Thurston's Philosophy of Marriage*

The author of the preceding asked a number of physicians the question: "Is sexual intercourse during pregnancy capable of causing,

a) Interruption of gestation (miscarriage)
b) Puerperal sepsis (blood poisoning)

The answer to this question was yes, invariably.

Many great men, including Chrishna, Jesus, St. David and Leonardo da Vinci, were born of mothers who did not live together, as wife and husband with their fathers. Chrishna's mother, during gestation, lived alone in the forest, subsisting entirely on wild fruit and berries. Mary, during her pregnancy, lived together with Elizabeth, away from her husband and from the father of her child. St. David's mother was a wandering nun, whose child was conceived by a king of a distant land. Leonardo da Vinci's mother, a peasant girl, lived apart from his father, who was of noble descent and who married another woman soon after his conception.

Plato and Buddha, like Jesus, were children of chaste gestation. Plato's biographer, Olympiodorus writes: *"An Apolloniacal spectre is said to have had connection with Perictione his mother, and appearing in the night to his father, Aristo, it commanded him not to sleep with Perictione during the time of her pregnancy, which mandate Aristo obeyed"*. After Buddha's conception, his mother lived alone away from her husband, in a special garden which was provided for her, eating only fruits and the products which nature provided. From that time no sensual desire ever disturbed her thoughts. She steadfastly obeyed, as she had done from her youth up, the Five Great Commandments, and abstained from all impurity, as the mothers of Buddhas ever have done.

The mother of Alexander the Great, during pregnancy, lived apart from her husband, Philip the Macedon. Since Isaac Newton's father died before his birth, and since chaste conditions prevailed for two years previous to his conception, we may assume comparative chastity during his gestation. Schopenhauer's superior intellect, like that of Plato's was due to a large degree to his chaste gestation, during which time his mother lived in a country villa, apart from her husband, who was engaged in business in a distant city.

Commentary by LIQUID METAL

'Pain' while giving birth to a child is not normal. When you understand and practice the information in this book, you should not experience any pain during and after the childbirth. The only normal pain that a human being should experience is if one is externally/physically hurt, such as when you fall, or when you bang the knee on a hard surface etc. Any emotional, mental and physical pain as a result of our ignorance, is our own doing.

There is cause and effect. The pain we receive is a direct result of the cause. Even if someone hurt us mentally or emotionally, it's also our fault for allowing that person to hurt us. Technically, nobody can hurt us mentally or emotionally without our direct/indirect permission.

PART VI

PAINLESS CHILDBIRTH

"It is well established by physiologists that the suffering attendant upon labor is abnormal, and only a result of violation of nature's laws; that by a more or less thorough compliance with these laws, most women can approximate a condition in which there shall be no suffering in childbirth".
– Dr. Stockham: *Toxology*/

"Pain in childbirth is a morbid symptom; it is a perversion of nature caused by modes of living not consistent with the most healthy condition might be counted on to do away with such pain". – Dr. Dewees

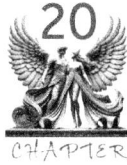

PAINLESS CHILDBIRTH THROUGH HYGIENIC LIVING DURING GESTATION

MAIA, THE MOTHER OF BUDDHA, when about to give birth to her child, walked off into the woods and while standing up, her son gently emerged from her womb, passing into the hands of one of her attendants. As a result of her vegetarian diet and her chastity during gestation (for she then lived alone in the garden), not only was her child painlessly born, but it came out perfectly clean, untainted by vernix caseosa. Jesus,

Jesus, as a result of his mother's chaste living and her vegetarian diet during pregnancy, was also born in a painless manner, without external assistance, emerging pure and clean.

Mohammed was painlessly born.

The mother of **Honen Shonin**, the Buddhist saint, as a result of her vegetarian diet, was free from sickness during pregnancy and pain during childbirth.

Confucius was born in a cave; **Apollonius of Tyana** was born while his mother was alone in his meadow; and **St. Francis** was born in a stable. In all the above cases, the mothers were not given drugs or anaesthetics, nor was the umbilical cord cut and tied by a physician or a midwife.

No woman is truly educated who does not know the hygienic methods of insuring painless birth. This knowledge will remove many groundless fears which are the results of ignorance and misinformation. As in the case of the animal, nature has constructed the human organism for the easy and natural accomplishment of childbirth. It is only the unhealthy and artificial life of civilized woman, and crude methods of medical interference, which makes childbirth as painful and dangerous as it is.

By chastity, natural food and hygienic living during gestation, childbirth will become an act of joy rather than of suffering, something to be happily looked forward to, instead of feared and dreaded. The first factor in insuring painless childbirth is continence (no sex, no masturbation, no orgasm) during gestation. Intercourse at this time, by irritating and inflaming the female sex organs, causes haemorrhages and pain during parturition.

"At one time, the author had a considerable experience with the Omaha and Pawnee Indians, and she studied these points with great care. She can most emphatically verify the forgoing, and furthermore can sustain the statement often made as to the painless confinements of Indian women. The natural delivery is severe muscular action, often, but not actual pain. Often an Indian mother has given birth to a baby in the afternoon and gone on the march the next morning. There is no denying the fact that the major part of suffering and discomfort of childbirth is due to sexual connection during gestation". – Teats, The Way of God in Marriage

The second factor in insuring painless childbirth is correct diet. Animal food such as, meat, chicken, fish and eggs, are poisons to the embryonic child, and should never be eaten. The diet should consist of raw vegetables, fruits and nuts. It is very important that the embryo receive sufficient organic minerals for the formation of its ductless glands and internal organs; these are more essential than proteins, carbohydrates and fats, which are more required during post natal development, when the child engages in muscular activity.

Dr. Cowan says: *"Pure blood being a requirement in the right growth of the child, it is almost unnecessary to say that a clean, sweet, lovable baby cannot be grown by a mother who uses fat meats, pork, spices, grease, tea, coffee, beer, whiskey, wine etc.; and even lean, fresh or healthy beef or mutton, the least harmful of flesh diet, are not fit to make babies of the right stamp. Undeniably, the best food for mother, during this period of pregnancy, is fruit and vegetables in as near to their natural condition as possible".*

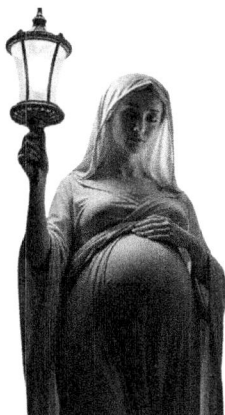

Dr. Stockham says: "*The fruit diet prevents the diseases of pregnancy and the suffering of parturition*". Ingestion, biliousness, headache, constipation, insomnia and vomiting during pregnancy, are to a great measure caused by wrong food. A pregnant woman in a perfect state of health, does not require any more food because pregnant than she would if otherwise.

Overeating during pregnancy causes the child to be extensively large, which leads to painful childbirth. A very large baby, encumbered with fat, is less healthy than a small one – contrary to popular opinions. The uterus, in which the embryo grows, is situated between the bladder and the rectum. When these are distended, it is compressed, and the growth of the child is inhibited. Therefore, overeating should be avoided, as this compression is liable to reduce the size of the embryonic brain. Laxatives or purgatives should never be used, for they are injurious both to mother and child. On a raw vegetable and fruit diet, they will never be required.

> **"**
> It is especially important to avoid the use of bread and cereals during gestation, if painless childbirth is to be insured. Not only are these foods not required, but they contain a great deal of inorganic matter which causes a premature ossification of the bones of the embryo, resulting in its difficult emerge. A too early consolidation of the bones of the foetus is one of the reasons for dangerous and painful childbirth.

LET GO OF TOXIC FOOD (PLEASURE) FOR LATER REWARD (JOY)

This in a great measure can be avoided, and the pain and labor greatly lessened, if the woman will, previous to confinement, abstain from. Graham or white flour, beans, peas, barley and all farinaceous substances, and milk, butter and cheese; in the place of these, using only fruit and vegetables. The child born under these conditions will be softer and smaller than usual, but will soon grow in strength and beauty.

Another writer says: "I was more particularly impressed with the importance of such a view, by the fact that in various parts of the world the females are comparatively free from the evils generally attending the females or European society. Among the Araucanian Indians of South America, a mother, immediately on her delivery, takes her child, and going to the nearest stream of water, washes herself and it, and returns to the usual labors of her station. Many accounts have been given of these and the females of other tribes requiring no more than ten or fifteen minutes for all purposes connected with delivery".

"In proportion as a female subsists during gestation upon aliment free from calcareous earthly matter, will she retard the consolidation of the child and thus prevent pain and danger in delivery. Hence the following may be given as an axiom for the guidance of females at these particular times. The more ripe fruit and the less of other kinds of food, but particularly of bread or pastry of any kind, they consume during pregnancy, the less difficulty will they have in labor. It is quite true to suppose that nutritious food is necessary to support and strengthen the foetus; but the nutritious and the solid earthly matter in food are very different substances. Wheaten flour, on account of its containing so much earthly matter, is the most dangerous article a female can live on when pregnant. The other grains are bad enough, but better than wheat" – Densmore, *"HOW NATURE CURES"*

Outdoor exercise, as involved in the gardening, is very important in preparation for a painless childbirth; and the easy confinement of Indian women is partly due to this reason. Deep breathing of pure country air is also essential, since the expectant mother breathes for two. The poisonous carbon monoxide of gasoline smoke is especially to be avoided. A daily cold bath is required; and also exposure each day of the nude body, particularly the abdomen and the breasts, to the sun's rays. (the ultra-violet rays, present at high altitudes, are extremely beneficial). Clothing should be light, loose and hung from the shoulders, wearing no woolen underwear, abdominal support, or anything tight around the waist or breast.

A woman who lives hygienically during gestation has no need to, and should never subject herself to vaginal medical examination. This crude and ugly practice (by which the physician puts his finger into the pregnant woman's vagina, pressing in upon the embryo from below as well as from outside) leads to injurious consequences both to mother and child. Continent and hygienic living during pregnancy will obviate all danger of foetal/fetal displacement or miscarriage, and no examination to know the exact time of delivery, nor in fact, will a physician then be necessary – Cowan, THE SCIENCE OF A NEW LIFE

Commentary by **LIQUID METAL**

In our current times, there is a lot of information and opposites of said information. For example, that Jesus never existed. Does it matter though? The meaning or message behind the information is what we need to focus on. Many times we have read stories (for example Zen stories) about life. Very good empowering stories. Does it matter if the characters in the stories were real or not? You could make up a story and give valuable lesson to a child that can benefit him throughout his or her life. The child won't care if it is real or not. But we adults on the other hand, we want something to be real according to what we think real is, because we are too stuck in physicality. We have been conditioned that someone in the story had to have been a physical person.

As long as you learn a thing or two from a story or a tale, then you can believe what you want, whether the main character or the characters of a story or a book (in the case of novels) was/were real person/people based on imaginative creativity story telling or from a true story. I had to explain about this because I know there is a big division among people whether Jesus existed or not. Also, another thing people argue about, is that his name was not Jesus but Yashua. Whether you believe his name was Jesus or Yashua, the belief is in direct proportion of your belief system. Wasting time about someone's name is like being happy to have found a shallow pond/river, while a little bit further (critical thinking) will show you the deep ocean.

Another not so bright arguing topic that I had the displeasure to listen to is about Buddha being fat. Buddha was an immaculately conceived superman; you cannot be fat when you are born perfect. In artworks, when Buddha is being depicted with a fat belly, it's about meditation. When you meditate deeply with the diaphragm, your belly swells. Try it, put one hand on your belly and consciously breathe with all your lungs (including the diaphragm) and watch how your belly will swell. Most people are shallow breather. Being a shallow breather, not only that millions of alveoli sacs in your lungs will become dormant over the course of your life, but you will use faster the number of the breaths programed you have in total over the course of the average life, based on your lifestyle. If we were (we can be) supermen or superwomen, there would be no limit to the breaths or the heart beats.

DON'T ALLOW GYNECOLOGISTS/PHYSICIANS STICK ANYTHING IN YOU. AVOID THE MANISTREAM CORRUPT HEALTHCARE SYSTEM LIKE A PLAGUE

Speaking of physicians sticking their finger into the pregnant mother's vaginas; that makes them perverts. For a healthy and intelligent child, a woman must only be seen and felt by the father of the child. Any other person, besides the mainstream healthcare perverts causing physical damage, but also energetical damage is caused. Any person carries in them energy residues from any other person they dealt in life, especially those who they damaged out of their ignorance or perversions in this case physicians who have inflicted a lot of bad karma by harming a lot of patients as a result of ignorance (or intentionally) for personal gain, as is the case when doctors receive bonuses when they get a certain numbers of new patients monthly.

Gynecology is seen as normal practice because it has been normalized and because it's legal. "Legality or illegality" are terms that enslave people's mind. Everyone of us carry the divine moral compass, we don't need the man-made laws to tell us what is right and what is wrong. Besides, the man made rules change over time. But the natural laws are unchangeable and eternal.

GIVE BIRTH IN THE COMFORT OF YOUR HOME

Following a vegetarian diet and chaste life (at least for a couple of years before conception until three years after the child is born), you can give birth to the child in the comfort of your home. Giving birth in a mainstream maternity, it is guaranteed that you and the child will be damaged.

Pushing the child out like most women do in the maternities, harms the child and the mother, it puts too much pressure on the child's brain and nervous system, let alone that the damage happens further when they cut the umbilical cord. But, just in case that you give birth to a child in a mainstream maternity, let the doctor cut the cord. Let him inflict bad karma on himself. Cutting the umbilical cord prematurely, is like physically hurting or killing a sentient being, you don't want to do that. Many people get bored in their own house. Because of that, they end up going in restaurant or other places or vacation. But when the temporary joy wears out, nothing has changed home. Make your home your vacation temple.

CHAPTER

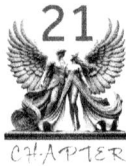

THE NATURAL METHOD OF CHILDBIRTH

WOMEN HAVE TOO LONG REMAINED IN IGNORANCE of the most elementary physiological facts concerning childbirth, which they have left to medical practitioners whose education, relating to this as well as to other matters, have been very faulty. As a result of this ignorance, both mother and child have been the sufferers. The high infant mortality today is sufficient evidence that the methods of childbirth now in vogue are unscientific, for they are largely based on superstition and tradition.

A woman should give birth to a child as easily as a hen lays an egg, leaving the process entirely to nature. This will be possible if she lives hygienically during gestation; childbirth will then be a simple muscular expulsion of the contents of the uterus. Childbirth is accomplished by the dilation of the neck of the uterus, and by the periodic contraction of the uterine and abdominal muscles, which cause the expulsion of the foetus. This occurs simultaneously with the bursting of the amniotic sac, in which the child, like a chick in the egg, lies enclosed. The head protrudes first; and finally the whole body emerges, attached by the pulsating umbilical cord to the mother. At the end of this cord is the placenta, which connects the foetus with the inner wall of the uterus, and which is expelled shortly after childbirth.

Two weeks previous to childbirth (which ordinarily occurs 280 days after conception) the premonitory signs of labor commence. By a softening and giving away of the os of uteri, the opening of the uterus into the vagina, and by a blending together of its body and neck, the womb sinks lower in the abdominal cavity, which results in easier breathing, and in many ways makes the woman feel lighter and better. A few days previous to the commencement of labor, the uterus sinks further (to the brim of the pelvis), resulting in an increased feeling of relief.

The first labor pains accompany the dilation of the neck of the uterus, to permit the exit of the child. The second labor pains, which are sharper and more frequent, occur when the muscles of the uterus commence their peristaltic action, expelling the foetus in a manner analogous to that of the rectum in expelling its contents. This expulsion requires no muscular effort, or "bearing down" on the part of the mother. Neither does the perineum need support. Dr. Stockham says: "A natural labour needs no manual interference. A Canadian physician asserts that he has attended 1,700 women in confinement without giving support to the perineum, and yet in no case did rupture occur".

When the child is born, it should not be immediately washed or oiled, but left to lie undisturbed by its mother. Its vital processes require time for adjustment to a new environment. It is not necessary that the child cry, which it will not do if it is kept warm and comfortable. The parturient woman requires no bandage. Anything tight around her waist after childbirth presses down upon the uterus and may cause prolapsus uteri. No clothing should be put on the newborn, nor should anything be wrapped tightly around it. If not prematurely cut, no tying of the umbilical cord is necessary.

"By tying, a small amount of blood is retained in vessels peculiar to foetal life. This blood by pressure or irritation may prevent perfect closure of the foramen ovale of the heart, and be a cause of haemorrhage. Besides, it must be absorbed into the system, causing jaundice and aphtha, so common in young babies". – Stockham, *TOXOLOGY*.

It is, unfortunately, a frequent custom to cut the umbilical cord immediately after birth. That is quite wrong, and may be attended with serious consequences both to mother and child. An hour should first be allowed to elapse; as soon as the cord is cold and the pulsation in it ceases. After a few days it falls off by itself.

Franz Anton Mesmer, the discoverer of animal magnetism, a physician, at first in Vienna, subsequently in Paris, says in one of his writings (A Warning Against the Premature Cutting of the Umbilical Cord): "It is the invariable custom, and has become an article of faith in all civilized countries, immediately in the birth of a child and before the placenta has made its appearance to firmly tie the umbilical cord in two places to prevent the loss of blood when the cord is severed.

With this hasty and violent treatment the circulation of the blood, shared by the mother and child, is suddenly interrupted without allowing time for the actual revolution to complete its circuit. The contraction and closing of the congested blood vessels of the mother, so necessary for the timely and natural delivery of placenta, is thereby prevented, and the latter is either torn off with more or less force by the midwife, or ejected by powerful contractions of the uterus. Injury to the interior of the uterus is the consequence, leading to haemorrhage, inflammation, tumors, suppuration, and more or less disease.

On the other hand, the blood contained in the portion of the cord · adhering to the body of the child, being withdrawn from the circulation, passes through every grade of decomposition on account of disturbances in the structure and functions of the liver. As a result, a subtle poisonous miasma is engendered, capable of injuriously affecting the liver and all bodily fluids".

Immediately after the birth of the child, its mouth and nose should be cleansed by the midwife. It should then be carefully covered and laid beside the mother until placenta makes its appearance. The child is born but the woman is completely exhausted by the demands on her strength and loses more or less blood (which ordinarily occurs, but not if she lives hygienically during gestation). What is to be done? Shall we follow the usual orthodox plan and allow the man to lose a large quantity of blood, of which she stands so much in need? Shall we abandon her state of weakness and wait the result? No.

"Haemorrhage after childbirth may be prevented, and thus the system may not be deprived of its needed blood, by the use of a cold hip bath. This need only take a minute. It causes a contraction of the uterus and a cessation of the haemorrhage. The placenta will then easily be expelled". – Bilz, *THE NATURAL METHOD of HEALTH*

If the mother lives a chaste and hygienic life during gestation, subsisting on raw vegetables and fruit, she may safely give birth to a child in the same way as apes and animals do, without external assistance or medical interference (which frequently does more harm than good). The umbilical cord would then be neither tied nor cut; it would be left to naturally wither away. When the child appeared, it would be brought into contact with the mother's warm body, and remain so as long as her intuition saw fit.

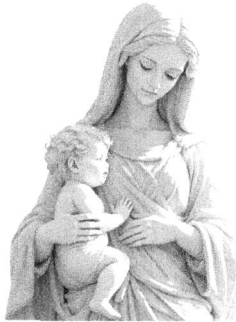

Difficult labour may be successfully managed without the use of instruments by means of hot sit baths. This causes a relaxation of the pelvic muscles (which are liable to be tense, because of the woman's nervous condition brought about by fear) thereby permitting an easier exit of the child, and reducing the pain. No drugs, anaesthetics or narcotics should ever be used previous to and during parturition, for it is better that the mother suffer pain (as a result of her previous wrong living) than that the child be poisoned (by the effect of the drug, transmitted first through the maternal blood and later through the milk.) Drugs also cause sickness and the death of the mother following childbirth. The 'milk-leg' after confinement is the direct effect of a large dose of ergot, a drug which poisons both mother and child.

"Pelvic peritonitis, puerperal or childbed fever, the death of the mother after childbirth is caused by:

First: The inflammatory condition of the system before delivery. If a fruit diet has not obviated this, there is nothing to fear.

Second: The use of ergot in confinement. Puerperal fever following poisoning by ergot is very rapid in its course and soon terminates in gangrene. If this drug were banished from practice, childbed fever would be rare.

Third: Contusions and bruises from instruments not handled dextrously.

Fourth: The use of cathartics, tonics, stimulants and other drugs after delivery.

It is within the power of every woman that she shall not be subject to these causes of puerperal fever. Instruments frequently maim both mother and child. Our statistics establish the fact that asylums are crowded with idiots and insane, who are so through the use of forceps in delivery. Through the use of forceps, the delicate unformed bones which contain the brain are maimed, flattened and bruised". Stockham, *TOXOLOGY*

Commentary by **LIQUID METAL**

Sometimes I have heard women say to men: "*Oh, you think it is easy to give birth to a child? I'd like to see you grow one and then give birth*". That is a negative low vibrational tone attacking men. While it is true that men cannot possibly know what it is to grow a child in the womb and then give birth through pain, the root of the problem is the unhygienic diet and sexual intercourse in general, especially while pregnant.

Men work in the most dangerous and filthy jobs that no woman would ever work at. What if men said: "*I'd like to see you work in those jobs, such as working 30 floors high in construction, or in the sewage systems full of filth/feces*". The beginning of the solution is to realize that we (both men and women) have been tricked and deceived into accepting their harmful practices, toxic food and drinks. We deserve and equally need each other. This corrupt and sick system exists because of the ignorant population. The sooner we wake up and create a bright, healthy and joyous lifestyle, the easier and faster the future generations will be rewarded.

Death of the mother or the child after the childbirth should not occur, there is no reason why the mother or the child should die. Nature doesn't make mistakes, man-made toxins and unnatural way of living is what causes the death of mothers or children after birth. Unless, the death is a result of some karmic bond, where the soul decided to leave, while the child was not born yet (miscarriage) or after is born, but that is another subject entirely. Here we are talking strictly about damage causes by us humans in this reality through carelessness and arrogance toward Nature and the Natural Law.

From unhygienic diet and sexual intercourse during pregnancy, not only that it harms both the mother and the child, for it will acidify the blood, but also women, most of the time choose an epidural which is injected right into the spine. Do you understand how dangerous that is? CSF – Cerebro Spinal Fluid flows in the spine. Through it, the Kundalini nerves will travel to the pineal gland. There can only be complications when you allow the mainstream healthcare system to inject poisonous substances in you. By choosing the epidural, it entices the woman to have more than one child. So, we (both sexes) have made mistakes over and over again throughout our lives so far. It is time to say, "ENOUGH IS ENOUGH". Let's begin a chaste and hygienic living step by step. If you don't remember, in one of the chapters there were eight steps. Find where you stand based on your current diet and work your way up the ladder of enlightenment and purity.

PART VII

INFANT CULTURE

"*We have evidence among primitive people that they understand the necessity of limiting offspring in a perfectly healthful way. The natives of Uganda, a region in Central Africa offer an illustration: 'The women rarely have more than two or three children, the practice being that when a woman has born a child she is to live apart from her husband for two years, at which age children are weaned'. Seaman, speaking of the Fijians, says: "After childbirth, husband and wife keep apart three or even four years, so that no other baby may interfere with the time considered necessary for suckling children*". **Dr. Holbrook,** *STIRPICULTURE*

"*And when three years expired, and the time of her weaning complete, they brought the virgin to the temple of the Lord with offerings*".
– *The Gospel of the Birth of Mary, Apocryphal New Testament*

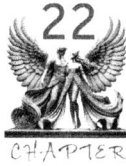

THE NATURAL LACTATION: FROM TWO AND A HALF TO THREE YEARS

IF A WOMAN LIVES IN CHASTITY, AND ON A NATURAL DIET during gestation and lactation, she (like all female animals who live in this way) will be able to nurse her young until their teeth have developed sufficiently to enable them to partake of their natural food. In the human being this normally occurs at two and a half years of age, until which time it should be fed on nothing but mother's milk. The giving out of the maternal milk supply at the end of nine months is an unnatural condition resulting from improper diet and incontinence during pregnancy and the nursing period.

The conception of another child before the natural weaning of the last one (which should take place as it approaches its third year) is harmful to the mother, the infant and the embryo. The mammary glands extract the most vital elements from the blood, thus starving the unborn child, while the enlarged blood supply to the uterus interferes with mammary secretions. Therefore, there must be no sex relationships for three years after childbirth, during which time mother and infant should live apart from each other.

Allowing a period of rest after lactation, and one of preparation before conception, there is a minimum period of five years between the successive births of children by the same parents. The sex act among married people, should therefore not occur more frequently than once in five years, and then only for the purpose of conception.

Observation will readily convince one that children who have had the advantage of being nursed throughout the period fixed by nature (from two and a half to three years) are superior to those whose lactation has been cut short at the end of nine months or before. The writer knows three sisters, all women of exceptional health, and mothers of gifted children who were nursed by their mother, an Australian peasant woman until they were three years old. Another woman who lived on a vegetarian diet nursed her child for two years, after which she raised it on a diet of raw vegetables, fruits and nuts (giving it no form of grain). The child, now five years old, is declared by educators to be physically and mentally supernormal.

Dr. Terman, the psychologist, after a recent survey of a thousand gifted children in the state of California, has come to the conclusion that superior mentality goes hand in hand with superior physical health, that the child of high intelligence has become what it is as a result of better prenatal and postnatal conditions, and that a greater number of supernormal children have been nursed by their mothers, and for longer periods than those of mediocre intelligence.

The cow is a stupid animal, with small brain capacity, and its milk is deficient in elements required for the adequate nourishment of the infant's growing brain. Therefore, a baby fed on cow's milk has a starving brain; its physical growth is overstimulated, but its mental growth is retarded. Mother's milk, since it is secreted from an organism with a higher brain-capacity (whose blood contains elements required for the nourishment of parts of the brain which are underdeveloped in the cow), properly nourishes the infant's brain; therefore, children who are nursed by their mothers develop superior intelligence than those that are bottle-fed.

The Prophet Samuel, like Mary, was nursed by his mother until his third year. Hannah gave her sin suck until she weaned him. And when she had weaned him, she took him up with her unto the house of the Lord in Shiloh; and the child was young. Since her husband had another younger wife, Hannah, like the mother of Mary, lived in chastity during gestation and lactation. It is a well-known fact that sexual intercourse during lactation induces premature menstruation, vitiates the quality and reduces the quality of the milk, and brings nursing to a sudden close. This results from the escape of genital fluid, which is otherwise lymphatically absorbed and carried by the blood to the mammary glands, stimulating their secretions. Genital fluid is very rich in phosphorus (as is men's semen), the element required to build brain-tissue; and a loss of it reduces the phosphorus content of the milk, retarding the brain development of the child.

The milk of the unchaste mother, like that of the cow, is deficient in elements required to build a superior brain. This is so because of her loss of seminal fluid (by orgasms and leucorrhea) and because of the resulting menstrual discharges. The dependence of the mammary glands upon this internally absorbed sex fluid is evident in puberty, when, due to an increased secretion and absorption of the latter, there is a rapid growth of the breasts, as well as of the brain and the entire body.

> **❝ SUPERMAN**
>
> Girls who masturbate, who are subject to losses of genital fluid, possess flat breasts. Menstruation is accompanied by the loss of this vital fluid, Hence, with its cessation after conception, the mammary glands commence to enlarge. As soon as menstruation begins again (determined by when sexual intercourse occurs), toward the end of lactation (which now takes place prematurely), the mammary glands diminish in size, lose their vital power and are unable to secrete good milk.
>
> **SUPERWOMAN**

Intercourse during lactation may lead to the poisoning of the infant by the lymphatically absorbed male seminal fluid, particularly if the father smokes or drinks. This male fluid, transmitted to the child through the milk, has the tendency to implant morbid sex impulses within it. Sex perverts and prostitutes are created in this way, as also through intercourse during gestation. It is a remarkable fact that the new-born of all other forms of life seem to have superior intelligence and ability than has the human infant, who, because of his larger brain capacity, should however, surpass them. This is due to the fact that the infant brain-cells have been paralyzed by its mother's unnatural diet and chastity during gestation and lactation.

There is no reason why, at birth, the cells of the brain should not be as fully active and co-ordinated as the cells of any other organ, such as the heart. Through hygienic and continent living, a mother may endow her child with a brain all of whose cells are functioning at birth. It has been estimated that most children are born with brains four-fifths of those cells are permanently dormant (having been impoverished, poisoned or paralyzed). This paralysis of the infant's brain-cells results in its typical stupidity as compared to new-born animals whose mothers live on natural food and in chastity during gestation and lactation.

Though it is universal, this condition is not natural. Children born from mothers who lived in chastity and on a vegetarian diet throughout their lives, as those of Krishna and Jesus, were reported to have displayed adult intelligence not long after their birth. This was due to the fact that their brains were nourished by sufficient maternal genital secretions (transmitted before birth through the blood, and after birth through the milk).

The growth of the infant's brain depends upon the concentration of genital secretions present in its blood (coming from either it's mother's or its own sex glands). This is illustrated by the following case of a child who had three sex glands, and therefore a greater amount of these secretions in its blood.

"At nine years of age this child possessed a fine beard and mustache, and had all the appearance of a young man of twenty. Short of figure, but very robust, he had strongly developed muscles and gave the impression of a vigorous man. His intelligence was equally far above that of an individual of his age. The parents, alarmed by the unusual aspect of their child, had the hypertrophied interstitial gland removed. Some months after the operation the beard fell out, the lad's muscles diminished in size, and which is still more significant, his intellectual development underwent a regression which brought the child back to a state corresponding with his age. We have in this case an excellent demonstration that the orchitic gland not only hold under their domination the factors connected with sex, but that they certainly act as general stimulant of our physical and intellectual energy".

Dr. Voronoff, from whose book, "The Conquest of Life", the above is quoted, contemplates the creation of a race of supermen by grafting sex glans into the bodies of gifted children. This suggestion is absurd, for if the child is supplied with sufficient genital secretions from the much larger sex glands of its mother, by her chaste living previous to conception, during gestation and during lactation, these same effects may be produced by healthy and natural means.

🕯 *Commentary by* LIQUID METAL

In this chapter when you read, *"there must be no sex relationships for three years after childbirth, during which time mother and infant should live apart from each other"*, that applies to fathers that cannot control their urges, men who are controlled by lust, men who need help because their weakness destroys them, the mothers and the children. But, when a woman and a man are living on a hygienic diet and chastity, then yes, they should be apart for three years after childbirth, because she could get pregnant (parthenogenic conception) just by man being present in the same place where she lives, only if he is the man where both their souls are connected. If you are a woman who lives a chaste and raw food diet lifestyle, you won't get pregnant if a man (who is not your partner/love, and who is also living the same lifestyle as you) walks by you.

If a man is controlling his urges, is not a problem if he stays with the mother of his child from conception until 3 years of the child's birth. As long as he doesn't cause her genital fluid to be wasted. Sometimes, the opposite sex partner (husband or wife) can turn you on so easily just be looking at him or her, where it causes you to secrete fluids. If that's the case, then the father should stay away from the mother, not necessarily in a different house or a city. If the house is big enough with a basement, then the man can stay in the basement. I know that it seems like a lot, but if you want to ensure that your child will be super healthy and super intelligent, you must create favourable circumstance for your child, or else don't have children.

Even if you are someone who wants to just have sex for procreation, you must live a hygienic food diet/lifestyle, because the cleaner your vessel/body is, the less times the man has to ejaculate. Nowadays, many couples try many times to conceive, which means too many seminal emissions and secretions from both the woman and the man, which means that an immense life force is wasted. If you don't have children yet, you are very lucky in these times where a lot of knowledge is available.

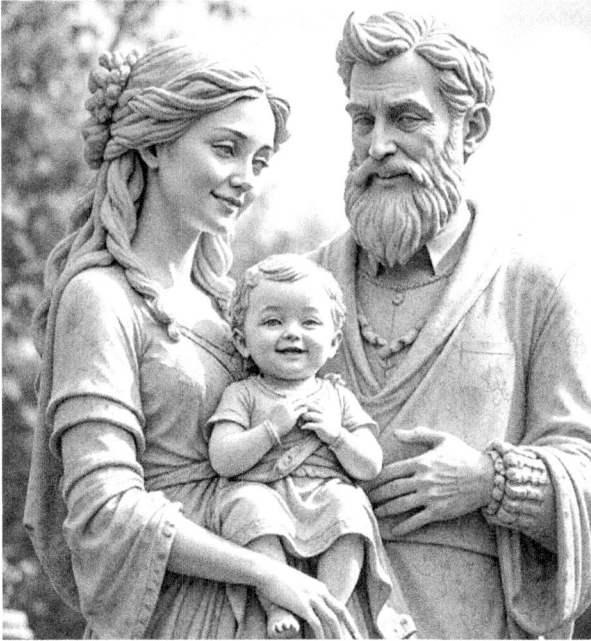

Decades ago, all I knew was, 'sex for pleasure' for many years. Just to conceive my first child, I had to waste my life force at least two hundred times, I was drained of it. It took me years to recover some of it. Please, consider the information in this book. You may be a meat eater or driven by lust and may ignore or disbelieve the rest of the book's content. This information is not an opinion. This book talks about the physiology and anatomy of mankind and how one can escape the prison of the body and mind.

Know that, if you stopped lactating the child shortly after birth or if you didn't lactate your child for at least two years, don't think that the child will be forever lacking. The child might gain what he lost, but a very big effort throughout his life is required. He must fast regularly, be on a raw food diet, connect with nature as much as possible, learn some kind of art. Even if we had billion of dollars to leave to our children, the money wouldn't all of a sudden make them intelligent children.

Knowledge and practice of it will turn someone into a wise man or a woman. When someone is wise, money will come, besides money should not be the goal; an open heart, a clear mind, high self-esteem, life force retention, gaining high spiritual faculties should be the goal, everything else is redundant. There is no reason why you shouldn't produce your own milk to feed your infant. Do not resort to store-bought formulas. They are poisons. Sure, they are good enough to not make your children become deformed where they have to build millions more hospitals for sick and deformed people. This system provides enough poisons as to not become an epidemic of a large scale. For example, the legal top speed on a regular highway is 80km/h (50 MP/h). There are just enough road deaths/accidents that it is not an epidemy. If the system could get away with setting the limit at 150, they would do it in a heart beat. The faster you drive, the faster you get to work, and also it creates possibility to work much farther from where you live. It would add more money/production to the system that would only enrich further those who don't care who lives or who dies. So, they have set the rules within a manageable rate. But this manageable rate is what it is because people have been desensitized.

A lot of deaths happen daily and people live their self-destructive lives as if everything is okay, and then they wonder why their life is a misery; they end up blaming the government, the freemasons, the Anunnaki, the reptilians or anyone else but themselves.

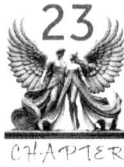

PSYCHOLOGICAL AND DIETETIC INFLUENCE DURING LACTATION

AS THE MOTHER MAY PHYSICALLY AND MENTALLY INFLUENCE the development of the embryo through her blood, so may she influence the infant through her milk. Nursing is a spiritual as well as a physical feeding; therefore, it is very important that every mother nurse her own child. If it is fed on cow's milk, it absorbs the animal qualities of the cow. If it is fed by a nurse, it will absorb her good and evil qualities. A mother who is not able to nurse her child should reform her way of living by eating simple, natural food and by conservation of genital fluid; she will then be able to nurse until it is old enough to eat solid food.

After the termination of nursing (between two and a half and three years after childbirth) the infant should be weaned and raised exclusively on fruit. Fruit will supply it with all the elements it requires for the formation of a strong, healthy body, even as grass supplies the needs of the calf.

The infant should never be given cow's milk. Cow's milk is unfit for human consumption for many reasons. Mother's milk forms small, soft curds which are easily broken up and digested, while cow's milk forms large, tough ones which are only adapted to the four-stomach system of the calf. Since the calf's period of infancy is only two months, cow's milk contains more rapidly maturing constituents which cause the child to grow at an abnormally fast rate. Babies fed on cow's milk may appear large and fat, but their tissues are not healthy. Cow's milk contains an excess of indigestible casein and lime, and a too small amount of milk-sugar and potassium. The most obvious difference between cow's milk and mother's milk is the fact that one is acid while the other is alkaline.

The infant is unable to digest cereal-starch in any form. Therefore, Zwiebach/zwieback bread, crackers and cooked cereals (or their juices) are injurious. Such food only turn into carbonic dioxide gas and alcohol, and are liable to cause convulsions. Water is not good for infants, whether boiled or not, it always contains a certain amounts of inorganic matter which may settle as calcareous deposits. Before weaning, the baby may obtain all the water it requires from its mother's milk; after weaning, from fruit.

The child, like the animal, should eat by natural instinct. When hungry, it should go to the food supply, and take the quantity and quality of fruit it requires. It should never be fed by its parents, nor forced to eat anything against its will (which perverts its nutritive instinct and is the main cause of children's diseases). A child raised on fruit will be physically, mentally and spiritually supernormal.

The thoughts and emotions of the mother, previous to and during nursing, through the glandular secretions which they induce, affect the chemical quality of the milk and the development of the child. These secretions, transmitted through the milk, will accelerate in the infant the growth of those organs, ductless glands and brain centers which have been most active in the mother, thereby reproducing in it the psychological traits she has then exercised.

During lactation, the mother should devote her time to the cultivation of the special talents which are to constitute the child's future life-work, which have been decided upon before conception, and which have been developed during gestation. The education of the child during the nursing period is more is more important than at any other time in its development (except for prenatal period) for its brain is never as sensitive to nutritional, environmental and psychological stimuli as it is then.

"Psychic conditions in the mother exert a powerful influence on the secretions of the mammary glands. Worry, grief, anger, fear and irritation not only diminish the secretion of milk but change its character and chemical composition, so that it may become distinctly injurious to the nursing infant. On the other hand, a pleasant and tranquil state of mind, combined with proper diet, will usually produce a copious flow of wholesome milk. Mothers should be especially warned against taking drugs and all kinds of stimulants during the period of lactation, for such

preparations will impair the quality of the milk and will often prove fatal to the child" – Carque, *NATURAL FOODS*

In the same way that the mother's habit of thought affect the child's character, so does the food she eats affect the child's physical growth and health, and, in a close manner, its mental characteristics. Especially during this period of nursing should the mother exercise the qualities (decided upon from the beginning) that in their transmitted action will constitute genius. After an intense application of brain-power in the direction required – be it that of mechanic, author, editor, teacher, singer etc. – the mother immediately following this application should give her child the breast. And precisely so in every department of childbirth.

A fat and heavy baby is generally the result of dietetic indiscretions on the part of the mother; the eating of too many cooked and concentrated acid-forming food; the extensive use of table salt, which leads to accumulation of water in the tissues of dropsical condition. Nearly all infantile diseases are directly caused by faulty nutrition and lack of hygienic care during pregnancy and the nursing period, and never by so-called infectious germs.

Of fifteen babies who die during the first year, only one is breast-fed. Overfeeding with boiled and pasteurized milk, the extensive use of artificial infant food, lack of fresh air and injurious prenatal influences are the principal causes of large infant mortality.

The newborn infant needs no artificial food. It should be put to the breast whenever it shows inclination. The true mother will delight in the privilege of nursing her child. It is highly important for the mother to be guided by and to protect the infant's inherent Nursing Instinct. The mother of young animals always has her breasts at their service, to which they go when they are hungry. The human mother should try to approximate this ideal. The only feeding schedule to follow is the infant's natural hunger. This, of course, necessitates the mother's continual attention to the child. Mothers whose minds are diverted by frivolities follow an artificial feeding schedule so that they may come to their babies only at certain times. But this is to the child's lasting detriment – for the human body is not a machine which may be fed according to the clock.

Commentary by **LIQUID METAL**

Humans are the only species to consume (not because they are thirsty or because nothing else is available) the milk of another species. Not only that people feed their babies and children with animal's milk but they themselves as adults consume milk and other animal by-products. It is simply brainwashing, consumerism at its finest.

Milk (dairy) is one of the greatest deceptions in the modern world. There are no animals drinking milk after weaning; and no, domesticated animals don't count. Milk, like many other artificial (or not for human consumption) food out there is addictive chemically. One of the proteins in milk is 'casein'. This protein may cross the blood-brain barrier and becomes 'casomorphin'. Casomorphin is also an opioid. Nature designed it to be addictive on purpose, so that the young mammals (animal or human infants) would enjoy nursing and come for more, until the three year requirement (for humans) where the brain needs all the important nutrients/organic minerals etc., so that then the child can be ready for solid food consumption.

Human milk has only 2.7 gram of casein per litre. Cow's milk has 26 grams of casein (morphine/drug). As we can see, this huge difference of casein between cow's and human's milk, tells us that milk is a powerful drug. Even if a cow's milk had the same grams of casein per litre as that of the human's milk, still, it should not be consumed by humans. It's mindboggling to think that drinking another specie's milk as an adult is natural. And even more mindboggling is to believe that it is natural to slaughter (even if you didn't slaughter the animal yourself, makes no difference) and consume animal meat a.k.a. dead, rotten and decaying full of pus and antibiotic flesh.

You must already know that there are a lot of nuts' juices where the word milk is used on the package and not the word 'juice'. Almond, walnut, cashews etc. liquids you purchase in stores are not milk but factory made juices. They are all harmful. Any product that needs to have a longer shelf-life, has chemicals inside. Even if it has a bit of real almonds or other nuts, it has been demineralized, processed to the point that it is a devitalized dead product. Just make your own nut juice. All you need is raw nuts, water and a mixer, that's all. You can add cinnamon or honey if you wish. It is much better to make your own than to rely on the toxic ones from the stores.

Making your own almond or any other nut's juice is also a way to transition from animal by-products to natural food and drinks. Don't think just because you may not have any discomfort in your physical body, it will continue to be that way. Any damage is accumulative, soon or later it will get you. We cannot escape the consequences of our actions. We cannot beat "time". Every present moment is precious. Be your own doctor, or else you might end up on the operating table one day.

When you live in low frequency state of mind (fear, worry, arguing, yelling, lying, lust, meat eating, alcohol and other harmful substance consumption, white flour, sugar and anything injurious mentioned in this book), not only that your milk would not be of the healthiest quality, but even if you are not having a child, your blood would by unpurified, your nervous system will become fractured, your seminal fluid would be depleted of nutrients, stem cells, phosphorus and organic minerals, your cerebro spinal fluid would not be of the highest quality for the purpose of activating you MERKABA; the Light-Body-Vehicle . I don't know who you are, but for me, when I first read this book (Dr. Bernard's work), I began to see health and life from a whole new perspective, even though I already had progressed a lot in my spiritual (mental, emotional, physical) journey.

THE SOLUTION TO THE ANSWERS ARE WITHIN YOURSELF

In our society you will hear the pregnant mother and/or the father use swear and/or sexual and perversive words. Anything that you say or think, rest assure that it will be transferred in the child. Even if you are someone who don't use bad (low frequency) words and/or thoughts, but you are in the presence of people (in the bus, train, mall, road or in general people you hang around with), your child will be affected for as long as you are within a few feet from other people. You already read in this book where many mothers of superman lived away from cities, away from chaos and poison. That's because they already knew that it would effect their child.

You may be a parent who may be wondering, "Why my child has turned this way, why doesn't he or she listens etc.? Assuming you are a role model parent, then the damage to the child has been inflicted from before he or she was born. Ask yourself these questions:

a) *Did I have sex while pregnant (or did I have sex when she was pregnant? - assuming you are a father reading this).*

b) *Did I have sex with her/him after the child was born?*

c) *Was the child nursed for at least two and a half years after birth?*

d) *Did I consume anything other than fruit and vegetables?*

e) *Did I smoke, drink alcohol, had sugary food and drinks?*

f) *While pregnant, did I ever breathed the smoking of other people?*

g) *Did I watch any movies/tv shows/You Tube or social media content where there was sexual content (visual, audible or written), politics, wars, or any talk that triggered me mentally and emotionally in a negative way?*

i) *Was the child's umbilical cord prematurely cut or was it allowed to fall by itself?*

j) *Did the child ever get any antibiotics?*

Answer these questions to yourself and you'll know for sure. But also, what if our children are smarter than us? We are conditioned to tell our children to obey authority. Parents are also a form of authority. There is a big difference between authority and leadership. When you lead your child to greatness, you are also able to admit your own mistakes when pointed out by the children. In a few cases I have heard both mothers and fathers telling their children to do something, and the children asked "WHY". The parent answered: "Because I'm your father, or I'm your mother". Well, that's not an intelligent answer.

REMEMBER THE CHILD IN YOU

First of all, children are curious being, and it's how it should be. Most people rush to grow up and then they get stuck in the adulthood lifestyle that is designed to keep them enslaved. Remember the childhood where there were no bills to pay, you were curious, you wanted to experiment with different things rather than living a boring and mundane life like most adults do.

We should feel good that our children have questions. Many parents are too tired from this system, where they have to work many hours and then when they come home, they are too tired to spend quality time with their children and so parents' emotional and mental state is so fractured that when children ask important questions that need to be answered by their parents in a calm and qualitative way, the children get shut down. It is true that you too as a parent have the right to be happy and free, but it is not children's fault. Bringing children in this world is a big responsibility.

Sometimes, yes, children may become annoying, simply try this:

"As a parent I know more than you, I brought you in this world. It is my responsibility to take care of you. But because I am your parent, doesn't mean that I know everything. When I tell you to do something, you have the right to ask me ONCE about the answer. And if I tell you do it a certain way, then you must do it that way. But as a being, if you have a different idea on how to do something, tell me, perhaps your way might be better"

The point is to communicate with your child, also this way you are allowing them to express themselves. If you shut them down, they might become pessimists and they might confide with other people things that they should confide with you. No matter how good hearted other people can be, you are the one that have a true bond with them, you would walk through the fire to save them if a situation like that occurred, nobody else would risk their life for your child as much as you would. Many parents unnecessarily have become enemies with their children because of lack of communication or heated arguments. That's what the Matrix' controllers want, for us to be enemies and hate each other. It's how they can easily manipulate us.

PART VIII

THE
EUGENIC
MARRIAGE

"Let the beam of a star shine in your love; Let your hope say: 'May I bear the Superman"

"Marriage: so call I the will of the twain to create the one that is more than those who created it. The reverence for one another, as those exercising such a will, call I marriage"

– Nietzsche: Thus Spake Zarasthustra

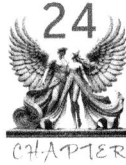

THE FOUR EUGENIC SANCTIONS PREVIOUS TO MARRIAGE

THIS BOOK IS TO BE GIVEN TO ALL CANDIDATES WHO MAKE application for Eugenic Marriage. They will be requested to carefully study it, and to reappear at a certain date for examination. This will be conducted as a psychological test, to be based upon the contents of the book. Marriage candidates who have successfully passed, it will be given **EUGENIC SANCTION NO. 1**

The candidates will then be given a thorough physical examination, by male and female diagnosticians respectively. If their state of health fulfills all physiological requirements, and if they are free from venereal, functional and organic diseases, and from injurious habits such as the use of tobacco, alcohol or drugs, they will be granted **EUGENIC SANCTION NO. 2**

Following this, they will be psychologically analyzed to detect their major abilities and talents, as well as their deficiencies. On the basis of this analysis, the unborn child's future lifework will be determined. This should be identical with the talents of the mother and with the parent's combined vocational aptitudes. Eugenic mates should be talented in the same directions. After deciding upon the child's future endowments, which are to be cultivated previous to conception and during the prenatal period, prospective parents will be given **EUGENIC SANCTION NO. 3**

Following the granting of this third eugenic sanction, marriage candidates are to go through a year's preparation for parenthood (conception), during which time they are to put into practice the principles contained in this book. At the end of this period or preparatory training, they are again to be examined, and if they show evidence of having lived the required hygienic life during the preceding year, they will be given **EUGENIC SANCTION NO. 4**, which entitles them to be eugenically married. This will be granted on the following conditions:

1) That they have lived during the preceding year upon a strictly vegetarian diet, using no alcohol, tea, coffee, tobacco or drugs.

2) That they have not engaged in any physical or magnetic sexual relationship during that time.

3) That they have cured themselves of seminal emissions, leucorrhea and menstruation.

4) That they have spent their time during the period of preparation cultivating the unborn child's future talents.

At the commencement of the period of preparation, marriage candidates are to be given a copy of the Eugenic Marriage Contract; and when they believe that they have fulfilled all necessary requirements, they will apply for the right to be married.

Commentary by LIQUID METAL

The word "Marriage" has lost it meaning. Nowadays, marriages happen between unconscious people. I speak from experience. I do not want anyone else to go through what I went through. Many marriages happen for all sorts of reasons, be it for personal gain or when the woman get pregnant by the unconscious man, although it's also her fault for having sexual intercourse with someone that she doesn't intend to have children. Many times, women trap men into marriage, that's because of the drive to procreate, but in the end, all lose, especially the child. Most men are driven by lust, this will eventually get them to go and meet women in the wrong places, and because the sexual organs are connected with the heart, many times men, or the women fall in love after they have had a sexual encounter, which will then most likely lead to marriage.

The description of marriage (Eugenic marriage) in this chapter, is how a marriage should actually happen. Not necessarily to receive certificates from some kind of agency but from a conscious and higher spiritual faculty state. But not everyone is capable to truly analyze themselves, so sometimes, guidance form others is required. Soon, more people will begin to raise their frequency and connect with their opposite sex on a conscious and soul level.

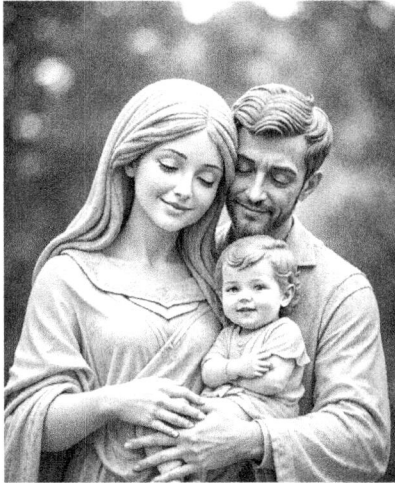

In condition #2, magnetic sexual relationship is mentioned. Which means that even if you don't have any physical touch with someone, even if you think about them in any intimately/sexually way, it voids the requirement to conceive a superman. But even if you don't believe, or even if you think is too much to let go (food, drinks etc.), fantasizing about someone will attract or lure spirits from the unseen realm toward you. And you don't know what kinds of spirits you will attract, most likely will be a spirit where when it was alive in a physical body, that person was attached to sex, alcohol, materialism, perhaps he/she was a narcissist etc.

It is a fact that many couples, when they have sex, they fantasize someone else, as opposed to being in the moment with the actual person they're having sex with. That's because there is no love anymore, boredom has numbed their senses. That's what happens when relations begin already in a decaying state, even though two people that get together don't realize it in the moment.

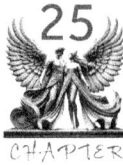

EUGENIC MARRIAGE

THE MARRIAGE SYSTEM OF THE PAST PATRIARCHAL AGE was based on protecting the sexual interest of men, while granting women a certain degree of economic security in event of childbearing. But it was anything but a eugenic system, and tended to promote race degeneration, instead race regeneration. In the New Age, marriage will be based on eugenic principles. It will no longer mean the selling by a woman of the nightly use or misuse of her body (more specifically her reproductive organs) in exchange for a home, clothing and food, but will have as its essential purpose the mutual desire of both parents to create a superman. The parents of Goethe married especially for this purpose; and the parents of Pythagoras and Plato dedicated themselves to the task of creating a superior child.

The economically independent and eugenically educated women of the future will be in a position to choose the best father for her unborn child, or better will produce one without a father, as did the mothers of Alexander the Great, Apollonius of Tyana, Zoroaster, Chrishna and Gautama Buddha. The initiative for conception will come from her, at the physiologically appropriate time, for she will have regained the lost instinctive sense of reproduction in relation to cosmic and solar cycles. The child will then not come into the world as an unwanted and accidental product of perverse sexual recreation, but as a work of art, prepared for during the course of years by devoted parents, willing to sacrifice personal feelings and desires for the sake of the coming Superman.

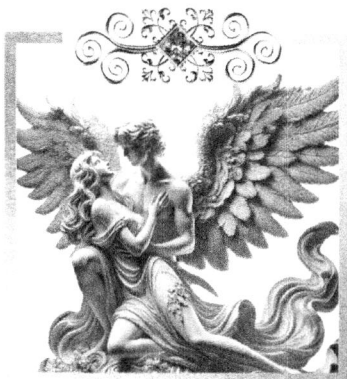

The new marriage ceremony will take the following form:

1) Do you promise not to conceive your child in the usual perverse manner, but either in the natural or in the immaculate way, by maternal initiative? (To be answered by both)

2) Do you promise never to engage in any form of birth control practices, or to conceive another child before the natural termination of the lactation of the previous one? (To be answered by both)

3) Do you promise never to commit abortion, or to permit abortion to be performed upon you? (To be answered by the woman)

4) Do you promise to live chastely, and on a vegetarian diet during pregnancy and lactation? (To be answered by the woman)

5) Do you promise not to engage in sex relationships with this woman during pregnancy and lactation? (To be answered by the man)

6) For what life-work has your child been dedicated? (To be answered by the woman)

7) What is to be the child's name (To be answered by the woman)

8) Will you develop your child's talent during gestation and lactation? (To be answered by the woman)

9) Do you understand how to insure painless childbirth? (to be answered by the woman)

Both parties are to retain their original names after marriage. The first name of the child is to be that of some great man or woman who has achieved distinction in the same work for which the child is being prenatally prepared; is surname is to be that of its mother. In front of the assembled audience, there should be a large painting or statue of this great man after whom the child is named.

Commentary by **LIQUID METAL**

Through the hygienic diet and chaste lifestyle period during gestation, not only that you can have a painless childbirth, but you can give birth to your baby in your home. There are more and more women in these modern times who give birth to their babies in the tub. Don't worry, the baby will not drown. The baby breathes through the umbilical cord. We have lost the ability to breathe underwater. One day, we will regain all lost abilities. All subjects here may be new and farfetched to many people, and it is understandable. How could someone believe that:

- *women can stop menstruating*
- *can conceive a child without the physical semen of a man*
- *men can contain their semen/life force forever*

We all have been brainwashed since birth that this man-made system is a natural one. And that is false. We are living in a corrupt decayed evil-man-made system. The ordinary method of child birth in mainstream maternities is terrorising, a butchery and it is a heartless practice.

AIM TO BE YOUR OWN BOSS

If you have two jobs, aim to work only in one. After, your aim should be to work less hours per day and finally until you don't have to work for a corporation. Opportunities to create income for yourself in the comfort of your home are endless. We are so lucky to have internet now. Do not live in scarcity mentality, because you will attract more of it. You must dislike your job so that you can make space for creating freedom for yourself and your children.

If a week had 10 days, rest assured that the government would make us work for nine days and give us a bone (one day off) to lick it. And if we have two days off a week, then that's two bones for us, meaning we still remain slaves with longer chains. A lot of people love their jobs, depending on the job, almost nobody works at a job that contributes into mankind's freedom. A friend of mine was an artist, nail polish artist, she loved her job until she realized that she was poisoning her clients. The nail polish disrupts the endocrine system, the lungs, the brain which interfere with the ability of a woman to sense truly divine/strong men's pheromones.

There is an abundance of money. The reason why people are poor is that the money that people spend goes into the pockets of greedy rich people. Instead of supporting the parasites who leech off the energy/life of humanity, support small business so that money circulates among us.

You may be wondering that what all these have to do with this subject. Any commentary by me has to do with the theme of this book. If people didn't live in scarce mentality, if people began to think for themselves, and take care of their body, mind and spirit, they would then become free, prosperous and live for a very long, if not become immortal. Immortality is for those who truly walk the path of greatness. In the path to immortality there is no room for laziness, passiveness, food/drink indulgences, untruthfulness, incontinence etc.

GOLDEN AGE

We are headed toward the Golden Age where our civilization will become fully conscious/connected with the Prime Creator or the Creation (depending on if you want to assign a noun/Creator or not). In the Golden Age people will be fully aware to the source within. Which means that we will realize that we are Gods and Goddesses.

Then there is the Silver Age. In the silver Age, people will need rituals to keep connected with the Source or the Prime Creator. It means that people are not connected anymore automatically from within, they need external reminders and/or internal as in the case of mantras or meditation.

Next, we have the Bronze Age. In this Age, mankind has lost its connection to the Prime Creator, or the Creators (people – Ex Gods and Goddesses). The creator/creators lose itself/themselves in the Creation.

Lastly, there is the Iron Age or the 'Kali Yuga', where humanity completely loses connection, where everyone is deprived spiritually, emotionally and mentally.

Some people are already fully connected to the Creation, but that doesn't mean that we are in the Golden Age. When majority is connected to the Creation/Creator from within, that's when it will be the Golden Age. Love and peace will reign in the Golden Age.

The length of an ascension cycle is about 25,920 years which encompasses four stages:

Golden Age (full LIGHT)
Silver Age (half LIGHT)
Bronze age (dim)
Iron Age (dark)

25.920 (the entire cycle) dividing by 12 zodiac ages = 2160. That's when the Golden Age will happen, in the year 2160. The year will be reset again, where we will go from year 1, 2, 3 until the next 2160th year before we repeat again.

Dont take this for a fact. Have in mind that the time is altered/ hijacked, or it is not, someone can be easily deceived by an obvious fact or by reverse psychology. As always, don't be lost in dates, names, calendars etc. When you feel too overwhelmed by information of the past or of what hasn't come yet (future), bring yourself in the moment. It is the only thing that can never be taken away from you. Every present moment is yours and yours alone. You are the master of time. But when you don't live in the moment, you become enslaved from it, not only that but others will use time on your behalf, but to their personal gain. Deep conscious breathing will always bring you in the present.

Years ago, when I heard that we would be living for 2000 (actually 2160 if the numbers are correct, but I guess people like to round up the numbers) in peace and fully connected to the Prime Creation, I would laugh and I would say: "Why not 5000 years, why not one million of years of peace, why not forever?" In my mind and in my heart I was right, but back then I had no knowledge of the full 25.920 (feel free to round up the number, it doesn't matter anyway) cycle. Now that I know, and this can be proven scientifically where we enter the Photon Belt half way through the Full Cycle. Higher spiritual beings would not give specific date to the masses. But I can guess the reason as to why they don't. That's because if they said that the Golden Age will arrive after 100 years, many people will become passive and lazy on their spiritual journey. I have already heard people say (when I mention to them about the Quantum Spiritual Medical Beds): "I want them to be available in my lifetime, I don't care about my next life time.

When you don't know the exact time when something happens, you are more inclined to learn/progress toward achieving something. Imagine if the masses knew that they would die next year or the next month, what would happen? Chaos of unprecedented proportion would happen.

In my mind The Golden Age won't happen for another 136 years, and yet I put this book together and I write a lot on social media and helping people with knowledge and wisdom in any way I can. Why is that? That is for two reasons, one because I'm driven by truth and love for mankind, and secondly, I know that we never die and that we reincarnate over and over again until we get it right, therefore fear, worry, lack of money, ungratefulness for my life, unappreciation etc. don't exist for me. When you get rid of the mental and emotional chaos all you're left with is "LOVE for everything deserving to be loved".

Be careful, numbers can trap you. Your subconscious mind takes everything as facts. If you think you are easily to be conditioned by numbers, then pretend that I said, "*We don't know when the Golden Age will be arriving, but what is a fact is that more light is coming in from the central Sun and we are ascending*". Some readers of this book may not know me, but some others that know me personally might take the number/year 2160 as a fact just because they trust my insight. Well, I say that "I KNOW NOTHING". Be your own researcher, historian, scientist, and doctor. Talking about dates is not insight but simply knowledge. It is important to not confuse knowledge with practiced knowledge (wisdom).

Don't forget that the Golden Age won't just suddenly arrive. We are in the transitioning period where more and more light is filling our bodies and the world. Picture a dark room, and then gradually turn the light on so that it gets brighter and brighter in the room. That's where we are now.

In the Golden Age, if money still exists, then it will be backed by precious metals such as, Gold and Silver. It is the only way for a balanced, and prosperous economy. Even if it will be a 100% digitally monetary system, the digital values of any country or the world, would still have to be based on the world's precious metal's value. Unless there will be invented another system entirely.

If this last chapter (I'm speaking of the Eugenic Marriage rules) causes discomfort in you as a man, either you reread the book and analyze yourself and the world, so that you may have an understanding of divine life where both genders are worthy to be equally free and respected, or for the moment focus on taking care of your body and mind, and then reread again the book.

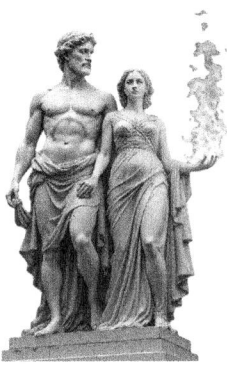

Patriarchal only society has been a failure. A matriarchal only society would also be a failure, but not as bad as a patriarchal only society. Unity between woman and man is the right balance. A cancer cell remains dormant until the person feeds the body with more poisons to the point that the dormant cancer cell will awaken and grow in size and take over the body. That's what happened in the distant past, were it was a matriarchal only society where the cancer (group of evil being, they were both men and women), a little at a time grew in size and took over mankind. Men were not strong, they were not poisoned because they were chaste and if they had sexual intercourse, they only did it for procreation purpose.

The point is that a strong man is needed in the Golden Age or any other Age. Not strong where he will beat and hit and destroy people and the world. Strong for themselves, for activities and to be ready to protect in case danger arrives, for example wild animals danger or saving someone when hurt and need help where muscle strength is required. The reason why I'm explaining about this is because there are people out there, especially some women who have developed hate toward men as soon as they were exposed to the parthenogenesis subject. Intelligence is when we don't only think about ourselves in this lifetime, but for all next lifetimes and generations.

If any information in this book triggers you in a negative way where it makes you want to defend the patriarchal masculinity idea/system, or if you are a woman that are trapped in the agenda that masculinity is toxic, you must try and see the bigger picture here. This is about freedom for all mankind. In the Golden Age, there is no place for hate, disrespect, deception etc.

At the end of this chapter (end of a chapter means before Liquid Metal's commentary begins) where it says that the surname of the child is to be that of its mother, it may angry a lot a men. If angers emerges, that's because of the patriarchal system of the last hundreds, or thousands of years. Let me ask you something, "Why are there no wars where soldier are all women?" You welcome. So, doesn't it make sense that if something in your life doesn't work, then perhaps it is time to change a new way of doing it?

The same applies here, patriarchal only society has brought wars, killings, raping, suppression of our society. If you are a man, know that the men of the world are not directly guilty. All men and women of the world want to live in peace, raise the children and enjoy a beautiful life. But those who enslaved mankind, had to choose men to go in wars and fight over an imaginary enemy. The real enemy was always the State/Government and organized religion.

In the NEW AGE (Golden) there will be no more wars, famine, rapes, killings, hate. Supermen and superwomen will reign this world.

Endnotes by LIQUID METAL

If you think that the current society's lifespan is normal, then you will not truly understand the importance of this book. We often dismiss information that goes against what's normal in our society. Normal is dangerous, it makes us passive and lazy.

1- Try and run for 5-10 minutes, if you can run without breathing through your mouth, then congratulations, you are beyond the average healthy.

2- If you are over 40 years young, try and jump and touch your chest with your knees/thighs while you jump, if you can do it, congratulations, you are not that unhealthy. If you cannot lift your own weight, that is a 100% indication that you are not healthy. Unless you had a surgery on your heap or knee and you cannot jump for now.

3- If you are over 40 years of age, on the floor stack about 10 books on top of each other, or anything that is about 10 inches (25cm) in height, sit on it, keep your feet and legs attached/close together and then try to stand up without using your hands/arms. If you can't, than it is a sign that you must lose weight, or even if you are not fat, you must walk, run and exercise to build stamina. If you build stamina, your body structure will automatically improve. If you are less than 40 and still can't get up, then that's bad. But no matter the condition of your health, you can heal yourself through fasting, exercising, sun gazing, sunbathing, grounding (meaning to walk barefooted on soil or on grass), raw food diet, meditation and preserving your sexual fluid.

4- Intelligence begins with how you take care of your body. No matter how many diplomas/degrees we have, no matter how many books we read, if we fail in taking care of our mind, body and spirit, we fail for good. Imagine if all life, everyone was raised on raw fruit and vegetables; and then someone came along and told you to eat processed food, processed drinks, alcohol, white refined flour/sugar products and countless of other toxic food and drinks, you would think that person is crazy for suggesting you such a thing. Well, in our society, people are poisoned so much mentally, physically and spiritually, where some call you crazy if you tell them that raw food diet is the way to be healthy. Most people's internals are graveyards. The digestive organs were not meant to become a sewage system but a link to the higher worlds/higher state of mind. Intuition in people is mostly blocked. Many are mentally swayed to do or not do things; to eat or not to eat certain food and drinks. But they think is their intuition. Intuition is not thinking, it is "feeling" the natural flow of the creation from your innermost being.

5- Do not fall for "Man is not needed to conceive a superman child". You just don't need his physical semen to enter through the regular method (sexual intercourse) that humans have been doing it for a long time. But you need his electromagnetism, his presence, his masculine energy so that all the parthenogenic conception process is applied divinely/naturally as intended, so that his electromagnetic force can fully awaken the X & Y chromosomes in both of you. It is a mutual process. Do not fall for the agendas that try to divide women and men, and causing them to hate and resent each other.

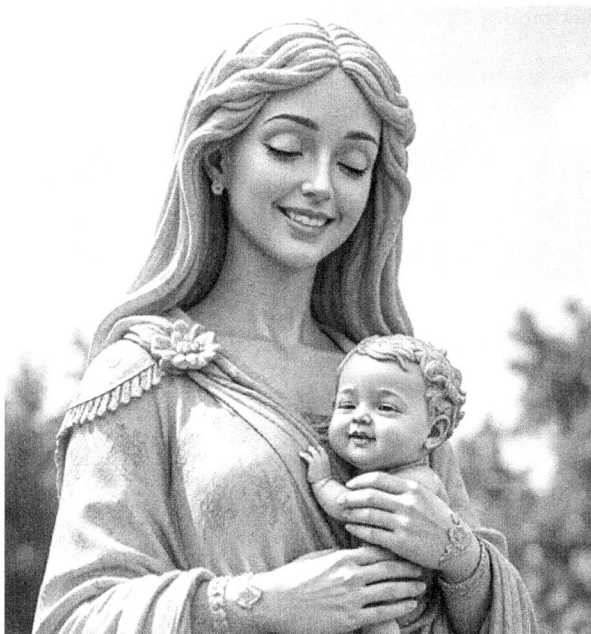

FURTHER READING/RECOMMENDATIONS

The Internal Dragon: The Art of Self -Mastery by J.J

To Be Reborn by Tamo A. Replica

You Are The One by Pine G. Land

Body Mind Soul by Saimir Kercanaj

Man's Higher Consciousness by Hilton Hotema

The Path To Greatness by J.J. and Tamo

Gain Wisdom Through Practiced Knowledge by Rimias K. Neo

DNA in the sands of time by J.Justice

I Am The Key That Opens All Doors by Saimir Kercanaj

Back To Eden by Jethro Kloss

Mainstreet Vegan by Victoria Moran

Juice Fasting by Steve Meyerowitz

First Water by Caraf Avnayt

The Chemistry and Wonders of the Human Body by George W. Carey

Food of the Gods by Terence McKenna

ABOUT THE AUTHOR

Dr. Raymond W. Bernard

Dr. Raymond Bernard was born as Walter Isidor Siegmeister. He was born in 1901 to a family of Russian non-practicing Jews in New York City. Later on he was known as Raymond W. Bernard. He was an alternative health advocate and esoteric writer, who formed part of the alternative health alternative reality subculture. Dr. Raymond is credited with the merger of the Hollow Earth theory and religious beliefs about UFOs. He passed away of pneumonia in September of 1965.

Some other books books by Dr. Raymond W. Bernard

Science discovers the physiological value of continence
Super health through organic super-food
Agharta The subterranean world
The serpent fire
From Chrishna to Christ
The mystery of menstruation
The revolt against chemicals